HEALING THE WOUNDS

HEALING THE WOUNDS

A Physician Looks at His Work

DAVID HILFIKER, MD

CREIGHTON UNIVERSITY PRESS

Omaha, Nebraska

Association of Jesuit University Presses

Grateful acknowledgment is made to the *New England Journal of Medicine* for permission to reprint parts of this book which were originally published, in slightly different form, in that journal. Chapter 6 appeared in the January 12, 1984 issue as "Facing Our Mistakes" (vol. 310, pp. 118-22). Chapter 8 appeared in the issue of March 24, 1983, as "Allowing the Debilitated to Die" (vol. 308, pp. 716-19).

Library of Congress Cataloging in Publication Data

Hilfiker, David.
    Healing the wounds : a physician looks at his work / David Hilfiker.
        p.   cm.
    Originally published: New York : Pantheon Books, c1985.
    ISBN 1-881871-23-1 (pbk.)
    1. Family medicine. 2. Medicine, Rural. 3. Physicians—Psychology. 4. Physician and patient. 5. Hilfiker, David. I. Title.
R729.5.G4H55   1998
610.69'52—dc21   96-47942
                                                                          CIP

EDITORIAL

Creighton University Press
2500 California Plaza
Omaha, Nebraska 68178

MARKETING &
DISTRIBUTION

Fordham University Press
University Box L
Bronx, New York 10458

FOR ROGER A. MACDONALD, MD

TABLE OF CONTENTS

ACKNOWLEDGMENTS

ANY PHYSICIAN WHO PRESUMES to write about his work owes a debt of gratitude to the patients who consent to having their "stories" made public. That debt is even deeper when the doctor is from a small town and his patients run the risk that—despite all attempts at camouflage—their own personal pain will become general knowledge. In writing such a personal book as this one, I expose not only myself but my patients, my clinic, and my community. I am most grateful for the encouragement and support they have offered me.

My physician partners and the clinic board of directors understood my need for the sabbatical that eventually resulted in this book. Despite the considerable inconvenience my leaving caused, they readily allowed me the fifteen months I needed for rest and reflection. I gratefully acknowledge their generous sacrifice.

I could not have afforded the extended leave from medical practice without the financial support of my parents-in-law, Martti and Elina Kaikkonen. Their offer of a place to live and rest, and especially Elina's provision of a quiet room in which I could write, made possible the initial work on the book.

Roger MacDonald and Gwenyth Lewis read the early drafts of the manuscript and offered their comments and insights. I have used their suggestions liberally, often without explicitly acknowledging my debt. It was their initial encouragement that gave me the confidence to proceed with refining the book and the determination to seek a publisher. Bill Gallea read a final draft from a medical perspective and made a number of helpful suggestions. I am very grateful to all three of these friends for their patience with me, and I freely acknowledge my debt to each one of them.

I thought I was finished with the writing of this book when I submitted it to Tom Engelhardt, my editor at Pantheon Books, but Tom gently guided me through the revision process, suggesting many improvements over the months we worked together. I am truly amazed at his ability first to notice changes that better the quality, and then, perhaps more important, to find ways to suggest those changes without offending me.

Finally, *Healing the Wounds* would have been impossible without the loving support, encouragement, and understanding of my wife, Marja, and our children, Laurel, Karin, and Kai. Perhaps it is never "fair" to ask a family to make the sacrifices of time and energy which writing a book entails; I can only gratefully acknowledge my debt to them and hope that they will get a little more of my time now that it is finished.

PREFACE
TO THE
SECOND PAPERBACK EDITION

HEALING THE WOUNDS was written in 1982 and 1983 about an experience of rural doctoring that began in 1975. Despite the enormous technological advances that have taken place in medicine since that time, the fundamental dilemmas practicing physicians face in 1997 have not changed much. The number of physicians and students who have requested copies of the book (which has been out of print for several years) is ample (and gratifying) testimony to its current relevance. I am grateful to Creighton University Press for their willingness to reprint this book.

When I first wrote the chapter on "Mistakes," I was completely unprepared for the reaction that was to follow. I submitted an early draft of the chapter as an article to the *New England Journal of Medicine*. Six months later (by usual standards a long time without any response), I received a call from Dr. Arnold Relman, then editor of the *Journal*. "Dr.Hilfiker," he began in his slow, sonorous voice. "We like your article, and we would like to publish it. But I must warn you that the publication of this article could potentially damage your career. You're young, Dr. Hilfiker, and something like this could close many doors for you. Please take a few days to think it over."

I will admit that his phone call made me a bit nervous. Was I naïve? Was I getting in over my head? But I read and reread the article, talked intensively to those that I knew might offer wisdom, and ultimately decided I had little choice: I had long ago made a commitment to truth-telling, and this submission to the *Journal* was simply a consequence of a choice already made. Besides. I thought I probably would have little interest in the particular doors Dr. Relman was referring to.

There were 150 Letters to the Editor in response to that article in the *Journal*, all but two of them affirming. In the thirteen years since that first publication, I have been stopped time and time again by physicians who have told me how important the article (which has also been reprinted in a number of anthologies) has been for them. They have gone on to say that the article gave them permission to forgive themselves and to be honest with themselves and their patients about their own mistakes; I have been told either in person or in letters many stories of their own mistakes. There are times when I feel that writing and publishing that chapter is one of the most important things I've ever done.

I find it interesting, however, that the attitude of the profession in regard to mistakes has changed hardly at all. In publishing I had seen myself something like the little boy pointing out that the King had no clothes and assumed that once articulated, the issue would obviously be important enough to warrant follow-up in the profession, that researchers or even physicians themselves would call for a change in the emotional milieu in which physician mistakes occur. But the silence has been deafening.

For many years there was literally no response: no follow-up articles, no categorization of kinds of mistakes, no study of the emotional effects of mistakes, no documentation of the pain suffered by physicians and their patients around the issue. Even today there are only a few articles; nothing essential within the profession has changed. Mistakes still have the same power over physicians they did in 1978 when I experienced the story I write about in Chapter Six.

It is fascinating to me that twelve years later most of *Healing the Wounds* is just as relevant as it was the day it was first published.

Certainly, ethical issues around the end of life have received a great deal of attention, and the dilemma I faced with Mrs. Toivonen in Chapter Eight would not be so confusing today. And it is also true that the physician's proper use of authority has now been written about extensively, but most of these writings have simplified the practice of medicine egregiously, suggesting that it is possible to simplify the relationship between physician and patient to a mere contract in which the physician has no real authority. The reality which every primary care physician recognizes is that our expertise gives us enormous authority and consequent responsibility, and we deny that authority at tremendous cost.

But most of the other concerns I address in the pages to follow remain still mired within the unconscious of the profession. That has surprised me, for I still believe that unless doctors experience deep emotional healing in the areas these chapters point to, we will continue to be haunted by them.

I hope the reprinting of *Healing the Wounds* will evoke enough interest to spark a reconsideration of some of the underlying themes: The sometimes necessity to be God, making life-and-death decisions essentially alone followed in swift succession by the need to enter into close person-to-person encounters or the mere banality of other meetings; the overwhelming emotional turmoil of a life so close to life-and-death issues; the uncertainty of actual clinical medicine in a world wherein the doctor is expected to be miracle worker. I have not seen other articles dealing with the ethics of doing insurance physicals on our own patients, the balance between efficiency and the art of medicine, and finally the morality of the high salaries available to physicians. These remain major issues within medicine that are yet to be seriously plumbed in any depth.

Nevertheless, much has changed in medicine. Seen from a contemporary perspective, the one glaring omission from the original printings of *Healing the Wounds* is the reality that physicians increasingly practice as employees of large, non-physician-controlled corporations and decreasingly on their own or as a part of a group of physicians run by physicians. (it was recently reported that more physicians are now employees of corporate bodies than work for themselves and there will soon be more physicians working for corporations than working in *any* other arrangement.) Although I have never had the experience of working within such a corporate structure, some of our patients in Washington belonged to Health Maintenance Organizations (HMOs), and I did have frequent occasion to deal with corporate medicine on their behalf, a task often onerous and frustrating.

I recall a minor example in which a hospital emergency room called me at home one weekend. One of my patients had come in because of abdominal pain; the pain was not severe, but the emergency-room physician was concerned about the possibility of appendicitis and recommended hospitalization for observation. I knew the patient and realized that her capacity for self-monitoring was minimal, so I also was reluctant to have her go home to be rechecked if things got worse. I concurred with the physician's suggestion to hospitalize the patient.

A few minutes later, I received another call, this time from the patient herself. Was I *sure*, she asked, that her insurance would cover this? Under ordinary circumstances, with ordinary insurance. I could have told her with certainty that since I, her primary care doctor, and the emergency room doctor both agreed on the importance of hospitalization, the insurance company would cover the costs of the admission. But the patient belonged to the HMO we had contracted with, and one of the iron-clad rules of the contract was that all hospital admissions would be cleared with the HMO itself.

I told the patient I would call the HMO and check back with her in a few minutes. I called the physician line at the HMO only to receive a recording that the office was closed for the weekend, recommending that I call back on Monday morning. I was incredulous! There was as far as I could tell no way that I could reach the HMO to have the admission certified.

I was quite aware that the HMO would probably certify the admission once I had explained the details, but could I guarantee that. No, I couldn't. It depended on which certifier I talked to and the precise language of a contract that I did not at that moment have access to. Knowing my patient, however, I was not about to give her another reason to leave the hospital and chance ruptured appendix. I called the hospital and without using the word "guarantee" was able to convince the patient to stay in the hospital overnight for observation. On Monday morning I called the HMO and did receive certification for the hospitalization.

It is, on the one hand, a mundane story. Everything turned out all right, and there was no damage. But it was a recognition for me that something drastic was changing. No longer was the decision about admission to a hospital in the hands of a physician and his patient; it was now directly in the hands of faceless "experts" at the (sometimes unreachable) other end of a telephone line. I considered the several times I had hospitalized a patient in Grand Marais for completely "extraneous" reasons (to get a woman out of a potentially abusive home, to give a tired-out elderly man a respite from taking care of his infirm wife while we made better arrangements, to reassure especially anxious patients that their sick baby would be okay). None of that would be possible under these arrangements; others much less intimately familiar with my patient would be checking on my decisions and determining their validity. Something fundamental within the doctor-patient relationship was changing.

I have heard stories of far worse intrusion into medical care, but for me the principle is clear from my simple example: While physicians must be continually educated about their fiscal responsibility, while irresponsible physicians must be disciplined, ultimately no third party should stand between the physician and his or her patient when medical decisions must be made.

The ownership of medical practices by for-profit corporations is as severe a threat to medicine and to the physician-patient relationship as we have known.

The current trend to corporate ownership of medicine began about thirty years ago with the advent of the Health Maintenance Organization (HMO) amid much hope of not only providing better health care but controlling the spiraling costs of medical care. By reducing the financial barriers to care and including preventive medicine as an integral part of all medical care, it was hoped that the overall costs could be reduced precisely because patients would be healthier. By organizing primary care and specialist doctors under one roof, it was also hoped that cost would be reduced. Finally, as part of the corporate body which "insured" the patient, the physician now had a financial incentive to keep excess costs under control and would make the decisions about what kinds of care were appropriate; the problems of excess testing and unnecessary procedures could thus be directly addressed. It seemed a wonderful solution.

But a number of our predictions turned out to be based on overly hopeful assumptions. Despite our prejudices, it turns out that preventive care (while certainly *better* care in the long run) is not necessarily less expensive than is acute care only. To give the most obvious example: A forty-five year old man dies from sudden death while shoveling snow. To save him from this fate through good nutritional counseling, expensive cholesterol lowering drugs, similarly expensive blood pressure control drugs, (to say nothing of the medical costs associated with the preventive care) only to have him die twenty years later from a cancer that requires expensive chemotherapy, multiple operations, radiotherapy, hospitalizations, and other expensive interventions might be much better for the patient in question, his family, and society in general, but it is not less expensive *to the insuring company* than no preventive treatment at all. From the point of view of company profits, it would be better if the employer paid the premiums and the man never showed up for any care whatsoever.

At the beginning of the HMO movement, doctors did not appreciate the potential for losing their independence once they became employees of a large organization. The possibility that significant medical decisions would be made not by physicians but by corporate managers looking at the company's bottom line occurred to very few of us, and—in our naïveté—we could not predict the limitations that would be placed on physicians once they became employees.

Doctors who for years feared the wolf of big government have left the backdoor open for the "grandma" of corporate medicine. "What a big mouth you have, Grandma."

Corporate medicine is the gravest danger facing the practice of medicine as a servant profession, and it is astonishing that organized medicine has not seen the danger and responded with all the force it possesses. I can only hope that this is the result of ignorance and not co-optation. If the organizations that claim to speak for medicine (and I'm thinking here primarily of the American Medical Association) will not lead the way in this, perhaps the rest of us (physicians, other health care providers, and patients) will need to become advocates in a much more political sense than we have previously seen the need for.

A second major development in medicine has been the gradual abandonment of the poor, both by medicine as a profession and by the society at large. Although the last chapter of this book explores this briefly, I have written in much more detail about the abandonment of the poor in *Not All of Us Are Saints: A Doctor's Journey with the Poor*. It is now clear that physicians' inability to maintain our commitment to universal access has been part and parcel of society's general abandonment and then active scapegoating of the poor. While there are still many rural areas (and even some small cities) where doctors have maintained the commitment to care for patients regardless of their ability to pay, those numbers are shrinking, and increasing numbers of Americans have no access to primary care.

The movement toward corporate medicine has also accelerated the medical abandonment of the poor. While there are many other issues involved in this abandonment, a physician employed by a corporation does not usually have the authority to allow into the office patients who cannot pay or even reduce the costs to what a person might afford. The non-paying patient never gets near the doctor; it's all taken care of at the front office.

From a spiritual point of view, the loss of this commitment to the poor has done irreparable harm to the medical profession, for it has made irrefutable the fact that the healing arts have moved from a servant vocation to become primarily a business. Shame for ourselves and for our profession coupled with a commitment to change is the only appropriate response. *Healing the Wounds* was written in a milieu which took for granted that any person needing health care would be welcome at our clinic and in our hospital. No physician I knew turned away patients who could not pay; no specialist I referred to even asked whether a patient could pay or not; no hospital I was associated with shipped or refused patients for economic reasons. We would have considered it unethical in the extreme. And that ethical reality has not changed despite our decisions to ignore it over the past twenty years.

I would expect, therefore, that certain elements of the book will appear naïve to young physicians. I would remind you that these expectations were obvious and unspoken as late as 1982 when I left northern Minnesota; in my mind the absolute commitment to provide medical care to all remains a clear expectation of a servant profession.

Once a book leaves an author's pen (or—in the case of the original version of this book—the author's mother-in-law's old Finnish typewriter), it takes on the status of the author's child, increasingly developing a life of its own. I must admit to some pride as I have watched *Healing the Wounds* grow and become a touchstone for many young physicians and other healers. I am grateful for the many non-physicians who communicated to me the importance of the book in their understanding their own doctors or, indeed, their own lives. The book is full grown now, and I'm happy to send it on its way again.

David Hilfiker, M.D.
Washington, D.C.

Chapter 1

CARDIAC ARREST

ROBERT MURPHY DOES NOT LOOK well. His left hand clutching his chest, he's in obvious pain, sweating, anxious. "It started almost two hours ago," he says, gritting his teeth, "and it took that goddamn ambulance forty-five minutes to get to our place. What the hell's going on? It feels like another heart attack."

It's one o'clock in the morning, and Diane Mattson, the night nurse on duty in our small county hospital, has just called me in from home. I'm still trying to wake up as I begin to question Mr. Murphy, who is lying on the emergency-room cart. Sixty-two years old, recently retired as the president of a small company in Minneapolis, he has just moved with his wife to our remote rural area for the summer. He tells me he had a heart attack five years ago in Minneapolis. His doctor there is a well-known cardiologist, whom he wants me to call. While I finish asking him questions and examining him, Mabel Wardly, the nurse's aide working tonight, puts an oxygen mask over Mr. Murphy's face to allow his heart as much oxygen as possible, and Diane inserts an intravenous catheter in his arm so we can give him emergency medicines if necessary. Diane then runs a cardiogram to see if he has indeed had a heart attack, and Mabel places him on the cardiac monitor so we can watch for any dangerous rhythms in the heart. Things proceed efficiently, and I am proud of Diane, Mabel, and our little hospital.

"What the hell is going on?" Mr. Murphy demands again. "I'm still having that pain. And what took that goddamn ambulance so long to get to our place? Did you call Dr. Johnson yet?" Mr. Murphy is scared and angry. I don't take the time to tell him about distances up here in the Minnesota

1

northwoods, about the difficulties of trying to cover an area larger than the state of Rhode Island with one ambulance.

"I'll call Dr. Johnson if we run into any problems, Mr. Murphy. Right now, though, we need to get you into a room and make you comfortable. Try to be patient with us."

Within minutes Mr. Murphy is in our coronary care unit receiving morphine for his pain and intravenous lidocaine to prevent a disturbance in heart rhythm so common and dangerous in these first hours after a heart attack. His cardiogram looks ominous: the picture of a serious heart attack. His rhythm is also becoming somewhat erratic, a clear sign of irritability in the heart muscle. I order sedation and add extra lidocaine to decrease the heart's irritability. I talk with Mr. Murphy briefly, trying to reassure him without lying to him. He is obviously frightened and no longer angry. Reviewing my orders with Diane, I tell her about my concern and ask her to call in a special nurse to stay constantly by Mr. Murphy's side until he has stabilized.

"Are you the doctor? I'm Carolyn Murphy. I drove up as soon as I could get myself together. How is my husband?"

I walk Mrs. Murphy through the halls into our cramped doctors' lounge, so we can talk in private. "Your husband's quite sick, Mrs. Murphy. He appears to have had a large heart attack, and his heart rhythm looks dangerous to me. He's in our coronary care unit receiving the attention he needs, but he's seriously ill."

She looks around at the bare walls of our doctors' lounge (actually an unused nursing-home room): a small desk, two folding chairs, a short row of old lockers, a single bed for night call. It's not very impressive. "Uh… don't you think we should transfer him down to Minneapolis? Dr. Johnson is his doctor there. We're…uh…so far away from everything here."

I take a deep breath. How many times have I tried to respond to this question in my years here? I'm tired, irritable. I don't feel like defending myself again. I want to go back to bed, but I can't leave this poor woman panicking in our small hospital. "We are far away, Mrs. Murphy; that's the problem. It's a five-hour trip to Minneapolis and two hours to the coronary care unit in Duluth. These hours following your husband's heart attack are the most dangerous. We just can't risk sending him in an ambulance at such a critical time."

"But can you take care of him here?" She looks at me, trying to find something she can trust. "I mean, I'm sure you're a good doctor, but…" Her voice trails off.

Mrs. Murphy's concern is certainly understandable. Who is this doctor, anyway, out here in the boondocks? I'm worried, too. I'm a family practitioner, not a cardiologist, and our two-bed coronary care unit is really only a regular hospital room with a cardiac monitor and some emergency equipment. Our nurses have taken extra training in coronary nursing, but that was two years ago; they can't be expected to have the same skill levels as the nurses in the big units in the city. I know Mr. Murphy is probably safer with us than taking the two-hour trip to Duluth, but I also wish he had had his heart attack at home where Dr. Johnson could attend him. Here in the middle of the night with an anxious spouse, however, is no time to dwell on my insecurities.

"I think we can take care of him, Mrs. Murphy. A lot of our summer people seem to come here to have their heart attacks, so we get plenty of practice. We've explored this question in detail with our consulting cardiologists in Duluth. They agree it's much safer to keep people here, at least during these first few hours. We don't have a sophisticated center like your doctor's in Minneapolis, but we'll take good care of your husband. I'm afraid you're sort of stuck with us. Your husband's in serious danger, and we simply couldn't in good conscience trust him to the ambulance ride right now. If you wish, we can talk about it in the morning after he's a bit more stable."

She looks at me again and takes the leap of faith. "OK, Doctor. I guess we don't have much choice, do we? But could you call Dr. Johnson in the morning?"

"Of course." We walk out into the hall, and I steer her to the waiting room. Mabel comes in with a cup of coffee for Mrs. Murphy and sits down with her.

I return to the nurses' station and finish writing orders. After reviewing Mr. Murphy's current tracings from the cardiac monitor, I step into his room and check him once more. Listening to his heart, I hear an S_3, an extra sound in the beat suggesting that the heart may be weakening. His lungs are still free of excess fluid, but I order a diuretic medicine anyway to keep the fluid from building up if the heart does begin to weaken. Returning to the nurses' station, I review the situation with Diane and Ardyce Millery, the nurse who has agreed to come in an extra shift to stay with Mr. Murphy. The heart rhythm has been stable on the lidocaine, but we'll have to watch carefully for complications. I decide to sleep overnight in the hospital so that a physician will be available right away if something happens.

It's almost three o'clock before I change into green surgical scrub-suit "pajamas" and crawl into bed in the doctors' lounge, but it still takes me an hour to fall asleep, and I sleep only fitfully. At five Ardyce knocks on the door: "Dr. Hilfiker, Mr. Murphy's having some irregular beats. Could you come take a look?" She opens the door a crack, and light spills into my eyes.

I get up, and we walk back to the nurses' station. "Is he having any other trouble, Ardyce? Any sign of heart failure?"

"No, that S_3 is gone, I think, and his lungs are still dry. Here are his rhythm strips," she says, handing me a series of tracings from the heart monitor.

I review them carefully. Mr. Murphy's heart rhythm has certainly changed. There are still some beats like those he had earlier, indicating an irritable heart muscle, but he also has another rhythm that is confusing to me. I'm not sure whether it indicates a worsening of the irritability or simply a minor malfunction of another part of the heart which wouldn't make much difference. How I wish I had a cardiologist by my side now!

"I'm not certain, Ardyce. I think these are only PACs with aberrant conduction, and we don't need to worry. Let's increase his lidocaine up to three milligrams a minute to decrease the cardiac irritability. Let me know if that rhythm gets any worse." I walk back to the doctors' lounge wondering whether I should do anything else. Should I try a more powerful medicine to decrease the irritability? Should I call in one of my partners even though I'm the only one on call? I close the door and drop back into bed.

For the next two hours my sleep is filled with dreams of monitors, Mr. Murphy's loud, angry voice, and imaginary knocks on the door. Just before seven the loudspeaker outside the doctors' lounge crackles: "Code Blue, room 2; Code Blue, room 2. Dr. Hilfiker, Code Blue." Mabel's voice sounds scared. I am instantly awake, stumbling by a chair as I sprint out the door in my stocking feet, around the corner, past the nurses' station, glimpsing Mrs. Murphy's desperate face pleading with me from the corner of the hallway into which she has retreated. I enter Mr. Murphy's room.

Cardiac arrest! The next hour flies by like a dream: Mr. Murphy's large body, naked, slightly swollen, bluish, lying on the bed; Ardyce and Mark Todd, the x-ray technician who's just arrived for work, expertly pumping on the chest and breathing into the mouth to perform cardiopulmonary resuscitation (CPR); the cardiac monitor's wildly irregular rhythm; Mr. Murphy's body jerking suddenly each time I administer electric shock from the defibrillator in an effort to start the heart again. The IV in his arm continues to flow, so I order another dose of lidocaine and two ampules of bicarbonate before I shock him again. Nothing. His heart continues to alternate weird rhythms I don't even recognize with a rhythmless twitching.

Ardyce is still performing mouth-to-mouth resuscitation when Mr. Murphy vomits, but she suctions him out and continues to breathe for him. Celia Warner, our anesthetist, arrives breathless from home and intubates the limp body, putting a tube into the lungs. All the time I am giving orders for medications, administering another electric shock, or asking for rhythm strips to see just how bad things have become. I try to maintain some clinical distance, to keep from getting too emotionally involved, to think clearly about what's needed next. I try not to remind myself that Mr. Murphy is dying. My mind enters another realm, detached, yet intently busy with the medical science of it all. The IV clogs, and Diane can't restart it; it's difficult to do when there is no blood pressure dilating the veins. A voice in the back of my mind wonders whether they have these kinds of problems down in the big city. Finally, Celia gets the IV going again, and we continue our medications, pounding on his chest trying to keep his blood circulating, breathing into his lungs for him. Once for half a minute Mr. Murphy's heart starts beating regularly on its own, and I hope against hope; but suddenly it's gone again, and we start all over.

I glance at Mabel, who is keeping track of the time, of medicine doses, of everything at once. It's been twenty-four minutes since he arrested. We've given him all the medicines I know how to give under these circumstances. There's nothing to do but continue with more of the same. The rushed panic of the first minutes changes into a steadier tempo. Celia inflates the lungs regularly; Mark Todd is back for his turn pumping on the chest to massage the heart; Diane administers IVS; two aides from the day shift run about gathering needed supplies. Mabel tries to catch my eye to read what I'm thinking. Through my mind run all the possibilities for therapy. Have I forgotten something? Is there anything else to do?

Suddenly time slows down. I realize it has been half an hour since Mr. Murphy showed any sign of life. His pupils don't react to my light any more. There is no spontaneous heartbeat when we stop CPR for a few seconds. I know his heart will not start again, yet I can't simply call off the resuscitation. Mark is pumping now on Mr. Murphy's chest, Celia is still forcing air into his lungs, the IV and medicines are still running. How can I just stop? In the back of my mind I remember those reports of full recovery after more than an hour of resuscitation. But not for Mr. Murphy! The rest of the staff avoid my eyes now, not wanting to appear impatient. I can sense the emotional fatigue in the room; they know it's become futile. I check his pupils once more: nothing. How do I decide there is no hope? I order another ampule of bicarbonate to give myself a chance to think. Is there anything else?

No.

Through my mind flash medical-journal articles on the definition of death. Much has been written by experts, physicians, ethicists, theologians. Who am I to take responsibility for saying there is no hope of recovery? Could there not be one chance in a million?

"OK, let's stop," I say. "He's dead."

No one wants to be first, but Celia finally releases her bag and pulls the tube out of the throat. Mark steps away from the body. I watch the heart monitor, fantasizing that the miracle of a heartbeat might reappear; then I turn it off. I don't want to watch the final flickers of electrical activity from the heart.

"Thank you, everybody," I say dully. "You all did a good job." I know how emotionally trying this sort of experience is for everyone. I want to support them, to encourage them, to be appreciative. But I can't do much; I feel in need of the support, the encouragement, the appreciation.

Walking out of the room, I am captured by Mrs. Murphy's eyes. She is silent as I walk over to her, sit down, and take her hand. I've never found a decent way to say this, so I just plunge in. "He's gone. We did everything we could, but he's dead. I'm sorry." I look into her eyes, trying to figure out where she is, how I can help. She knew already, of course, but the finality of my words brings out the tears. We just sit silently, my hand on her shoulder, both of us exhausted from the night. There is really nothing left to say, but I'm uncomfortable without anything to say or do. Finally she looks up at me with all those questions in her eyes: Would it have helped to get him here earlier? Would it have been better in Duluth? Was everything possible done for him? Why couldn't you save him? But all she says is, "I suppose I'll have to fill out some papers." I sit with her a few more minutes, describing some of what happened to her husband, but— numbed by the sleepless night, absorbed in her own grief—she isn't listening.

Finally, I leave her in Diane's gentle hands and walk to the doctors' lounge. I know I'm going to be late for my hospital rounds and my morning appointments at the office, but I sit here for five minutes anyway as the emotional impact of the last hours washes over me. Familiarity with death does not, in fact, remove its sting. No matter how inevitable death may be for each one of us, a patient's death always seems like my personal failure. "We did everything we could…" My words to Mrs. Murphy echo through my tired mind. Why did I say that? Was it to defend myself against her unstated accusation, was I denying my own uncertainty, or was I just trying to comfort her, to assuage the guilt that always follows death? I don't even know for sure. All the decisions race through my head again, and I wonder what I could have done better. Should I have tried to transfer him to Duluth? Should I have stayed up with him myself, given stronger medicines? Should I have asked my partner to come in? Could anybody have saved him? Why do they always seem to die? There are no answers, of course, and there seems to be nothing I can do with the feelings that burn inside me.

As I get up to return to the nurses' station, I notice the charge sheet on the desk. What do I charge Mrs. Murphy and her insurance company for unsuccessfully attempting to keep her husband alive? How much is it worth? Do I charge less than if I had succeeded? Is the money supposed to ameliorate the feelings of guilt and inadequacy I'll face over the next few days? Will it make my kids happier or make up for my bad mood when I finally get home tonight? Somewhat bitterly, I decide not to think about it and only write on the sheet: "Attempted resuscitation—ninety minutes." I'll let Mirna try to figure out from her code books at the office how much to charge.

I walk numbly back to the nurses' station. I have four patients in the hospital whom I need to visit, office hours begin at nine, and it's already eight forty-five. I pick up my first hospital chart, but then notice Ardyce sitting in the corner by the sink, tears running down her cheeks. I put my hand on her shoulder as she looks up. "I'm sorry, David. I should have called you earlier, but I wanted to let you sleep. It all happened so quickly. He was just talking with me, asking how he was doing, when he passed out and the monitor alarm went off. We called you right away. He was so scared....It's never happened to me before." She lowers her head, and I can feel the tears welling up in my eyes, too. We're both exhausted. Ardyce has to come back to work the three-to-eleven shift, and I have an office full of patients waiting. When do we deal with our emotional pain?

■

Eventually the pain became too much. This book is the story of how that happened to me and what I tried to do about it; but it is also the story of many other doctors, perhaps even of many other helping professionals: of the conflicting pressures they face, which often seem to defy solution, and of the responses they come up with, which often become problems in their own right. It is by now one of the world's most poorly kept secrets that anxiety, depression, loneliness, and burnout are major factors in the lives of many doctors. Nothing could have convinced me more of this than the hundreds of letters I received from doctors all over the country and in all different kinds of practices in response to two articles I published in the *New England Journal of Medicine* on the issue of doctors' mistakes (my own included) and some of the ethical dilemmas in medicine. I sensed in these responses the powerful desire of doctors to speak honestly about the problems of their professional lives and the pressures they face every day for which neither the structure of their profession nor society at large in any way equips them. Typical of such letters was this comment from a Dr. Roth who works in Oregon:

> Thank you for articulating feelings that I, and I feel many other physicians, have but are too insecure to express. In the past three years two very competent physicians committed suicide in our relatively small medical community. Both men were in their forties with families and a great deal going for them. I suspect that somewhere in their psyche they had experienced the turmoil that you expressed in your article—the inability to free themselves from the yoke of perfection that our role of physician has imposed upon us.

While this is very specifically a book about my experiences as a family practitioner in a small town in northern Minnesota, I wrote it with an awareness of the rising tide of criticism against physicians as a group, criticism of our attitudes toward patients and of our general behavior. We are accused of being unavailable, of no longer making house calls, of being scheduled weeks in advance, and of hiding behind telephones and receptionists. We are too preoccupied with disease and not concerned about the whole person. We don't listen to our patients, won't communicate with them. We are authoritarian, dictatorial. We are told that we place too much reliance on science and technology, and that we don't put enough energy into personal, caring contact with our patients. And we're too interested in money. Our prices are impossibly high, our incomes extravagant. "Doctors don't really care any more. It's just a job to them."

There is truth in all these allegations, but they do not go far enough. As I write about myself, I also see the signs that doctors as a group suffer because of their work. The statistics are stark: the United States loses the equivalent of seven medical-school graduating classes each year to drug addiction, alcoholism, and suicide.[1] Physicians tend to be workaholics. Even intact families without obvious maladjustment suffer from the physician's progressive emotional separation from family life.[2] Both patients and physicians seem to be suffering.

Although this is not a sociological study of physicians, my personal struggle is hardly unique. Many prospective doctors, I think, come to the first year of medical school as basically well-adjusted, highly idealistic young people. (I remember clearly the murmur of disapproval that ran through the audience of beginning medical students during our opening ceremonies when an older physician began describing the "good life," the material rewards of the physician's career. *We* were not there to gain prestige or money but to alleviate humanity's suffering.) The same pressures and contradictions that drove me temporarily from practice also drive other idealistic medical students into the seemingly uncaring behavior of many later careers.

When I am in the midst of caring for a Mr. Murphy, there is little time or energy to dissect the multiple stresses that assault me. Everything happens at once in a confused and confusing barrage. However, on reflection, the stresses seem to divide themselves into two general groups. In the first chapters of this book I want to examine those which seem to be built into the nature of a doctor's work. The extreme intensity of medical practice and the need to be constantly available to patients (even in the middle of the night) creates a background level of tension from which the practitioner can rarely escape. The impossibly broad range of knowledge necessary to daily practice (from taking care of heart attacks to delivering babies), the ever-present uncertainty in diagnosis and treatment, and the ubiquitous possibility of making life-threatening mistakes are brutal emotional facts of the doctor's life. We are faced continually with ethical dilemmas for which there seem to be no solutions. Despite our oath to act on our patients' behalf, we are often pressured to act as society's agents against the interests of individual patients.

As difficult to deal with as these are, there is a second kind of stress which, though less obvious, undermines even further the doctor's ability to do his or her job well, no less to believe that that job is "worth it." We physicians, like many other professionals, have accepted certain values, certain ways of behaving, which run counter to the very basis of our profession—the ideal of service. The emotional distancing that may initially be necessary to medical evaluation comes to dominate the physician-patient relationship. We allow ourselves to accept certain standards of efficiency and productivity which militate against caring for our patients. We accept positions of prestige and authority which separate us from our patients and co-workers. And we have never resolved the contradiction between our high salaries and a career of service. To a certain extent these values, too, are structured into our very work; yet it is helpful, I think, to look at them more as responses to the first group of "built-in" stresses. We physicians usually perceive these responses of clinical detachment, efficiency, prestige, authority, and wealth as helping us to deal with the pressures of practice. In fact, as I will argue, they become a problem in themselves and only make things worse. If it is possible to deal with the stresses of medicine, I believe it must be done by restructuring our work around some other values. The last chapters of this book are my own exploration of what this might look like.

Although I believe that most of what I have to say is applicable to any physician employed in the primary care of patients, this book is basically an attempt to understand the nature of my work as a rural, family-practice physician. My situation in our small clinic was probably even a bit calmer than that of many other rural doctors. Our clinic in northern Minnesota, more than 110 miles from Duluth, the nearest large city and referral center, provided the only medical services to a county of over 1,300 square miles of woods and water. Nevertheless, we had an adequate number of physicians to serve our population of 4,000 permanent residents. When I arrived I joined two other physicians, and a few years later we added a fourth partner. Our office was initially a satellite clinic in a federally subsidized experiment in rural health care administered from another city in Minnesota, 150 miles away. When the large distances between the satellite clinics and the administrative center proved too cumbersome and impractical, our community received further federal grants to administer the clinic as a community-controlled, nonprofit corporation. Thus, we physicians were never burdened with many of the administrative and business functions that other physicians (who own their offices and run their "businesses") must carry. We were free to concentrate on our medical work.

As the only physicians for sixty miles in any direction, we were responsible not only for the clinical care of our patients but also for most of the other medical needs of the county. Located on the outskirts of town, our office was set slightly apart from the rambling brick structure that housed the county's hospital and other medical services. One hundred feet from our clinic door was the hospital's emergency-room entrance; directly inside, the emergency room for which our clinic physicians provided twenty-four-hour on-call coverage. When the county population swelled from 4,000 permanent residents to over 20,000 people during the summer tourist season, the emergency-room practice became a major element in our work.

Just southwest of the emergency room was the newer nursing-home section of the hospital complex, where we provided care to about forty-five elderly residents; southeast was the old wing where we would walk by a jumble of rooms—the laboratory, x-ray suite, small operating room, delivery room, waiting area, and administrative offices—before coming suddenly into the sixteen-bed hospital itself: eight patient rooms lining one side of a long hallway with the nurses' station at one end and an old laundry, now used as an outpatient alcoholism treatment unit, at the other. This old section had been built in stages, apparently without an over-all design, and despite its small size, a newcomer could easily get lost in its hallways, which turned repeatedly upon themselves. It was my home for seven years.

Our town was a wonderful place to live. The business area was small and clean. The surrounding residential district melted gradually into sparsely settled country and then into a rocky wilderness of birch trees and pine forests and scattered lakes. From our house high on a hill, I could run the two miles to work at the clinic and hospital during the warm weather and ski back and forth on cross-country ski trails during the winter. The townspeople allowed us physicians our individuality and with certain exceptions respected our call schedule, generally accepting our need to live our own lives. I worked with partners who were compassionate and competent physicians, with whom I could share a practice; and for a clinic organization that allowed us to develop our own schedules while it recognized our need for time away from our jobs.

None of this saved me from the pressure cooker of the job itself. As the crises and the all-systems overload piled up, my initial reaction, like that of many doctors, was to try to devise various technical stratagems that would give me room to maneuver, room even to breathe. I cut back from a sixty- or seventy-hour work week to one of forty-five hours, and we added a fourth partner so that our call schedule would be more reasonable. That helped a little, but my unhappiness grew. I next assumed that it must be my own fault, so I entered into a counseling relationship with a most understanding therapist and spent a year and a half exploring the sources of my discontent. That helped too, for, as I hope will be only too clear in this book, I have my own hang-ups and they are an integral part of the story. But I hope it will be equally clear—as doctors' responses to my earlier writings have made evident to me—that there are deeper causes than my own dissatisfaction and unrest for the problems I faced and tried so desperately to cope with.

This book is intended for people on both sides of the medical experience. Although I have tried to use non-technical language and to explain certain medical phenomena in lay terms, I hope that other physicians will not let this put them off. For those physicians who are interested in thinking about the stresses of their own lives, I hope this book will be of some assistance. For medical students who are not yet wrapped up in the structures and values of medicine, I hope it will provide inspiration to create a more humane alternative for their careers. For other medical personnel who must work daily with physicians, I hope it will stimulate compassion and encourage cooperative efforts; physicians may need some prodding from you to create new structures. And for interested patients, I hope this book will give some insight into their doctors' worlds, thus allowing new relationships to begin. Finally, although this book is about the particulars of the medical profession, I hopé some will perceive the fundamental alienation inherent in our male-dominated technological society and will glimpse some possibilities for change.

Before I begin, a few comments are in order. I am writing about the life of a rural family practitioner because that is my experience. Although the particular stresses of that life may be unique, I do not wish to imply that they are worse than those experienced in other vocations. On the contrary, since many of them have to do with the way we structure our society, it would be my hope that other helping professionals might find in these pages illumination for their own lives.

Quite frankly, I do not know what to do with the English grammar rule that says we must use the pronouns "he," "his," and "him" when we mean to refer simply to a person of either sex. The continuous use of the masculine pronoun distorts reality. Given the current stage of our language, however, I know of no comfortable alternative. Borrowing from Gordon Cosby's usage in *Handbook for Mission Groups*,[3] I have generally elected to use both feminine and masculine pronouns: when the physician is "she," the patient will be "he," and vice versa. It is my hope that the reader who notes his or her own discomfort with this usage will take some time to ponder the reasons for that discomfort.

Finally, the stories I use as illustrations are all drawn from my experience in practice. The dialogues attempt to render conversations as best I can remember them, but they are certainly not verbatim transcriptions. In a few cases I have merged two or more separate events into a single story either because I couldn't remember exact sequences or because the combination of several stories helps to illustrate several points simultaneously. Most of the stories, however, are as accurate retellings of what actually happened as my memory will allow. By using the personal stories of my patients in a book like this, I risk exploiting unethically the confidentiality with which I have been entrusted. I have of course changed names and details, but certain stories are impossible to camouflage adequately, especially in a small town. In these cases I have shown the manuscript to the patients involved and received their explicit permission. The enthusiasm with which they encouraged me to pursue this writing has given me the courage to take that risk. I am grateful to them for their willingness to share of their lives.

Chapter 2

THE PRESSURE COOKER

IT IS A THURSDAY in the fall. Tourist season is over, the leaves have fallen, but the air is warm with the return of a brief Indian summer. Today is my day on call: in addition to my regularly scheduled patients, it is my turn to see those without appointments who walk into the clinic, to cover the emergency room in the hospital, and to be available during the evening and night for anyone in the county who needs medical attention. I should be well rested and ready for the demands of the day, but I was up much of the night helping a baby to be born. Although the delivery went well, I am exhausted and that makes me irritable. Fortunately, the office staff recognizes my tiredness and is pampering me. Jackie Mullen's job as receptionist today turns into an ongoing attempt to protect me from an overload of patients, a thankless task.

The morning goes remarkably smoothly. There are only a few walk-ins and I begin to think I'll last through the day. Shortly after I begin seeing my afternoon patients, however, Marge Armundt, the nurse who usually works with me, interrupts a prenatal examination to tell me that the ambulance has just been called out to one of the wilderness resorts. A small boy fell into one of the countless lakes in our area and was pulled out; someone is performing artificial resuscitation while awaiting the ambulance. No other details are available. It will be over an hour before the ambulance can reach the scene and bring the child back. There is nothing I can do to help at this point, so I return to the examination room and my pregnant patient.

Ordinarily, I enjoy these prenatal visits. In a schedule crowded with sickness and discomfort, they are an opportunity to talk about health with patients who are excited about their condition. I can relax and enjoy the relationship. But now I have trouble concentrating on the questions she is asking me. Half of me is with the ambulance, wondering who the child is, what his condition. It is difficult to be in two places at once, but I can't just cancel my afternoon's patients. I pay attention as best I can.

My next patient is fifteen-month-old Troy Johnson, crying listlessly in his mother's arms. Bonnie tells me Troy was fine last night but woke up this morning with a 104-degree temperature and has been cranky all morning. I ask some more questions and examine him carefully. Aside from his fever and listlessness, however, there are no specific findings to indicate a diagnosis. He probably has an early viral infection. I explain to Bonnie what I'm thinking and suggest that she watch carefully for signs of dehydration over the next day or two.

Bonnie seems relieved. "I thought it was probably just a virus, but our friends' little boy down in St. Louis just died from meningitis, and I was scared. I just wanted to make sure."

Meningitis! I haven't seen a single case in the five years since my internship, but early meningitis is a possibility in any young child with a fever, even if the physical examination seems normal. And Troy's listlessness would fit. The only way to know for sure would be a lumbar puncture, an expensive procedure in which a fine needle is inserted in the lower back to remove for testing a small amount of the fluid that circulates around the spinal cord and brain. It is pretty traumatic even for a fifteen-month-old, to say nothing of his mother. We were instructed in our internship that if we even thought of the possibility of meningitis we should do a lumbar puncture, but I see two or three children like Troy every day: I can't tap every child with a fever! All I say to Bonnie is, "I don't think it's meningitis. Keep a close eye on him, and if he gets any worse let me know right away." She is satisfied, and I decide not to share with her the small chance that Troy may indeed have meningitis. I reiterate the things she should look for, but keep the doubt to myself. For the following two days that tiny possibility will bob repeatedly into my consciousness, setting me slightly on edge.

As I finish dictating my notes on Troy, Marge tells me that the ambulance has arrived at the lake and is picking up the child. It is Ricky, the four-year-old son of Tom and Joan Meier. No one knows how long he was in the water, but John Hempsted, their next-door neighbor on the lake, pulled him out and started artificial respiration right away. The ambulance crew is continuing CPR, but there's no word on Ricky's condition. It doesn't sound good.

"Has anyone contacted Joan?" I ask Marge. Joan is a patient of mine, a teacher at the school. She and her husband own a resort and manage it full-time while working at other jobs to make a living. I can't imagine the agony she is experiencing as she waits to find out what has happened.

I call over to the hospital to make sure the emergency room is fully ready and the staff will be there to handle whatever situation presents itself. I review what we might need to do, how to prepare myself. My adrenaline is already flowing, and it is difficult to wait for the ambulance.

My next patients are in the examining rooms, however, so I try to be attentive to their stories. Fortunately, their problems are straightforward. I can handle them satisfactorily even with my mind continually straying to the ambulance and its cargo. As I begin dictating on the second chart, Marge informs me that the ambulance has radioed in. It's five miles out of town. I walk over to the emergency room.

The siren comes wailing down the hill. The ambulance pulls in to the rear entrance between the clinic and emergency room and backs up to the door. Jack Huber scrambles out of the driver's seat and opens the rear doors of the ambulance; I can see Maurie Dickerson, the ambulance attendant, and Linda Stapleton, the emergency-room nurse, working methodically on the boy. I marvel at Jack and Maurie: they both hold down full-time jobs in town but are on twenty-four-hour call every other day to respond to emergencies like this one. At any time, day or night, I can call them and they are available, frequently for the six-hour trip down to Duluth and back. Our small-town medical care system depends on their dedication.

Ricky is quickly hoisted down from the ambulance and into the emergency room while Maurie and Linda continue cardiopulmonary resuscitation. The boy is blue, his limbs flaccid. I remember newspaper stories about young children pulled from cold northern lakes after even forty-five minutes who survive to live normal lives. Two other nurses from the hospital relieve Linda and Maurie at CPR while others strip the boy of his clothes, attempt to warm his body, and attach the heart monitor. My role is simply to direct the action, but I am deeply involved. Is there anything we can do to save him?

The heart monitor shows a flat line—no spontaneous heart activity. Jack Huber gives me as much of the story as he was able to get at the scene. No one saw Ricky fall into the lake or knows how long he was there. John Hempsted was at the boy's side as soon as he was pulled out and started CPR right away, but no one has seen any signs of life. The ambulance crew continued working the entire way down to the hospital, but Ricky has now been out of the water almost an hour.

I turn back to the boy. The hour in the warm air has warmed his body, but his pupils do not respond to the light I shine into them, his heart shows no sign of electrical activity, and there is no spontaneous breathing. I see no point in continuing the resuscitation. I tell the nurses to stop CPR. I can barely look at Jack or Maurie or Linda; they have given themselves to that kid for an hour, trying against all odds to save him, and I've pronounced him dead. The ambulance crew and the nurses mill about the emergency room for a few minutes, not knowing what to do. Someone pulls a sheet over Ricky's body, and people leave one by one to return to their routines.

Linda comes back into the room to tell me that Joan is in the waiting room. Someone called her over from the high school. I try to switch gears emotionally, to change from the detached clinician in charge of a technological intervention into a compassionate human being, a friend who cares, a father who can share a mother's grief. I too am overwhelmed by the tragedy; I consider my own children safe at home and wonder briefly how I would respond if it were one of them lying on the table.

The waiting room is only a large alcove off the hallway between the nurses' station and the emergency room, so Joan has certainly seen the staff running back and forth as we have worked on Ricky. She has also seen them retreating slowly back to the nurses' station, so she must know he is dead. No one will have told her directly, of course; tradition and etiquette reserve that task for me, the physician, even though many of the others are Joan's friends too.

I sit down beside her and put my arm around her shoulders; as she looks up into my face it is easy to read the anguish of the last hour. "Ricky's dead, Joan."

She nods her head and covers her face with her hands. "He was dead when they pulled him from the water, wasn't he?"

"I think so. Nobody noticed any signs of life. John got to him right away, I guess, and the ambulance crew worked on him all the way down to town, but I think he was dead already." I have nothing to say, no medical wisdom or profound words of consolation, so we just sit. Joan and I are not close friends, but we know each other well enough. There's no need to say much. People walk quietly by. Joan is still; her tears have stopped for a while.

"Does Tom know?" I ask her.

She nods. "He's on his way down. He'll be here soon."

"Do you want to go in to see Ricky?"

"I don't know...I'll wait until Tom gets here. Maybe we'll go in together."

"OK." I become aware again of the patients waiting for me over at the clinic. I am torn between wanting to stay here, just to sit with Joan, and my feelings of responsibility to those who have appointments. Which is more important? Feeling vaguely guilty, I stand up and ask Linda Stapleton to sit with Joan while I return to the clinic. There is hardly time to take a few deep breaths before I am back in my examining rooms.

"Dr. Hilfiker, I just don't feel right any more." Mrs. Sophie Williams sits slumped in her chair in the corner of the room, looking at the floor as I enter. Only sixty years old, she appears eighty: obese, anxious, depressed, in terrible physical health. Mrs. Williams's remaining joy in life seems to be complaining. She visits the clinic regularly, seeing first one doctor for a couple of months and then another as she discovers we can't help her very much.

"My back has been bothering me again, Dr. Hilfiker, and I can't get no help from nobody. Nobody cares for me. Can you help me? If you could just help me get some sleep at night. Dr. Masterson used to give me pills to sleep at night, but you young doctors don't believe in helping an old lady sleep, do you?" She looks up at me, her grin incongruously punctuating her lament.

I take a deep breath and sigh. I feel a churning inside. On a better day, I know, I could empathize with Mrs. Williams's pain, with her emptiness. I could sit with her, take an interest in her back pain, talk about her sleeplessness. I could encourage her to talk for a few minutes about her loneliness, about her anxieties. And she would leave feeling a little better simply because I'd paid attention. But today isn't a better day. I'm tired, grieving over Ricky's death, concerned for Joan. I try to pull myself together, force myself to empathize, but it doesn't happen. I can't find the energy. Mrs. Williams gets nothing from me today. As she leaves, I hear her talking with Marge: "I wish Dr. Masterson was still here. At least he cared about an old lady's sleep."

I reach for the next chart in my box. It is brand-new. I scan the personal information: Anne Wilson, thirty-four years old, recently moved here from California with her husband. Clipped to the outside of the chart is Marge's note: "Wants Valium." The churning inside begins again. I've never met Mrs. Wilson, but I can guess what the next twenty minutes is going to be like. She's just about to incur a $23.50 doctor's bill to be told that she won't get Valium from me. "My doctor in California always gave it to me whenever I needed it," she will tell me. "I don't abuse it, but I need it to relax." And I will try to be patient and tell her why I prescribe tranquilizers only rarely and then only temporarily. Finally, she will leave the office angry with me and with our clinic. I take Mrs. Wilson's chart and walk slowly back to my desk. Sitting down, I bury my face in my hands. I'm not sure I can take this today.

■

Very little of my work as a physician was glamorous in the TV drama sense, but much of it was intense. Daily I was tossed from sore throat to heart attack, from psychosomatic illness to life-threatening emergency, from birth to death. Each patient required my full emotional involvement, my full energy. Even an apparently minor illness could bring an unexpected challenge, for serious illness or injury can lurk behind any seemingly innocuous symptom. I had to be constantly on guard. I could be sitting at home in the middle of dinner only to find myself, several minutes later, trying to prepare a severely injured accident victim for safe travel down to the referral center in Duluth. Even a routine delivery could in no time at all turn into a nightmare, involving the resuscitation of a newborn baby or desperate attempts to stop bleeding in the mother.

As a primary care physician I was not always on the edge of crisis. Indeed, weeks would sometimes pass between "exciting" cases, but the hazards were always there. Routine heart attacks or asthma attacks may not have the obvious thrills so many of us have been trained by television to expect of doctoring, but each may take that unexpected and sudden turn, and thus each required my close attention to any signs that could possibly indicate danger. Indeed, even mild illness in the very young or the very old spelled possible danger, for in such frail bodies any illness might suddenly destabilize.

As a result, it was my job to be thinking of the worst complications that could happen. Every child with a fever could be a case of meningitis; every adult with unexplained weakness or weight loss, a potential cancer victim; every stomach ache, a possible appendicitis. Since, in addition, medicine is so inexact, I could rarely know for sure. Every patient called for my full attention. My job was to take each illness with the utmost seriousness.

To further complicate this picture, most patients perceive the illnesses they bring to their doctor as serious. Medical sociologists know that a primary reason for consulting a physician is fear that symptoms may hide some important illness. "Fearful persons," one physician has written, "are fatiguing and unpleasant to work with and their fear is often contagious.... [Medical practice] consists in routinely interacting with persons who are anxious, uncomfortable, and often unable to express gratitude or affection."[4] Even when I've discovered quickly that a symptom is benign, it may by no means relieve the intensity of an encounter, for the patient still remains to be convinced, often a more difficult job than making the original diagnosis, and requiring skills I was never taught.

I was, then, constantly on the firing line. Every moment required the utmost vigilance. But I was also expected to act normally, to be reassuring and calm. Mrs. Williams, for instance, needed my full attention. There was no opportunity for me to deal with the smoldering feelings left over from Ricky's drowning, to tell her I needed an hour off to deal with my grief. I was immediately swept on to her problem and then on to the next.

Almost more difficult to deal with was the internal roller coaster that mirrored the outer swirl, each external event leaving its own indelible emotional imprint. As I think many doctors discover, it is simply not possible to respond adequately to the ongoing intensity of such situations; I was left wondering whether I should have done anything else before halting Ricky's resuscitation attempt, whether I could have been more comforting to Ricky's mother, whether I should have waited for Tom to arrive before returning to my office appointments. Since I hadn't really dealt with my grief over Ricky's death, or had time to face the very human sense of inadequacy the total situation sparked off in me, I was hardly able to deal with Mrs. Williams's problems...which, of course, only made things worse. Even as I tried to sort out everything else, one part of me was very aware of giving second-rate care to Mrs. Williams.

The emotionally healthy life requires a balance, a certain rhythm for moving back and forth between crisis and routine. As a physician, though, I rode continuous roller coasters, both outer and inner. There was simply no occasion to digest what had happened, to think about it, discuss it, integrate it into my life history. The only way I found to cope was to harden myself to it, to shield myself from it. This skill of detaching oneself emotionally was inadvertently taught to us from the beginning days of medical school. Each of us, for instance, spent our initial several months dissecting a cadaver, a dead human body, in the necessary process of learning human anatomy. Before we entered the dissection rooms for the first time, our nervousness and tension were evident. Would we be able to handle it? Would we get sick? What did it feel like to make the beginning cut? The first day or two of dissection were somber, serious. We knew what we were doing: cutting apart the physical remains of a human being. Within weeks, though, the mood changed completely. Each cadaver gained a humorous name. Jokes passed from table to table. Discussion centered on the evening before or next week's test. The reality of dissection could not be endured, so we protected ourselves from it, built barriers between ourselves and the existence of our cadavers.

That very same process repeated itself daily in our medical careers. The first year in medical school, for instance, can be seen as a process of learning a new language: medical jargon. Heart attacks become "myocardial infarctions"; cancer becomes subdivided into countless varieties of lymphomas, carcinomas, disseminated metastases, and terminal illnesses; even poverty is transformed into a "psychosocial complication." Much of this jargon is absolutely necessary since the vernacular is simply not refined enough to bear the complexity of medical knowledge. Necessary or not, however, the jargon distances us physicians from our patients and from the reality of their disease. The names give to the diseases a rigid definition, a cleanness, belied by real diseases in real patients. By the end of that first year of medical school, we knew the language, and we had been initiated into a role which required a certain distance between ourselves and our patients. At the end of that first year, we were also taught physical examination and diagnosis. In order to learn the technical skills of examination, we practiced initially on each other. In our group of five students, there were three men and two women. This quite naturally caused some embarrassment as we came closer to the days when we would practice breast exams, genital exams, and rectal exams. I remember asking the question of our instructor, "How does one handle one's own feelings of sexual arousal when examining someone of the opposite sex?" His answer was essentially that those feelings should not arise, that they should be suppressed as completely as possible. Even as a student I knew that would not be possible. I sensed a deep unwillingness to have us look at our own feelings.

As we moved into the years of clinical practice, the intensity of what was happening around us was simply too great. To protect ourselves from the horrors of the emergency room or intensive care unit, we discovered the grisly jokes of the medical wards. The elderly, terminally ill, toothless patient who lay with mouth rounded for better breathing was said to show the ominous "O sign"; if the patient deteriorated further, and the tongue hung from one corner of the mouth, it became the "Q sign," indicating imminent death. Patients who were difficult to manage because they complained of an excessive number of symptoms (many of which were probably caused by severe emotional distress) had long been labeled "crocks," so that even the emergency-room nurse would warn us before we entered the room that "a real crock" awaited us. It was not long before one intern amused everybody by requisitioning a "serum porcelain level" from the lab to determine objectively whether the patient was indeed a "crock."

Within the space of several days, one of my fellow interns had two emergency-room patients whose hearts stopped exactly at the moment he was listening to their chests; both patients died. For weeks afterward the other interns referred to his stethoscope as his "deathoscope."

The jokes, the names, the apparent callousness, may seem shocking to the outsider; for us—to the extent that we had occasion to reflect—they were simply ways of protecting ourselves from the intensity of our feelings. Patients became "cases"; persons became "strokes" or "MIs" (medical jargon for heart attacks). To say "There's an MI in room 1" was clearly a step in shielding ourselves from the reality of our patients' anguish and pain.

Every physician discovers that doctoring offers many opportunities to retreat from the intensity of the medical experience. Exaggerating the required clinical detachment, busying oneself with efficiency and productivity, hiding behind the profession's prestige and authority, entering into subtle competition with other physicians to prove one's competence, or earning as much money as possible all provide avenues for separating oneself from the overwhelming nature of each day. But this is not the only pressure that leads to the creation of such barriers. The necessity to be almost continuously available may be worse.

Chapter 3

THE LIMITS OF HELP

FINISHING MY HOSPITAL ROUNDS and walking back toward the nurses' station, I glance at my watch: 8:55 A.M. I have five minutes before I'm due at the clinic. "Wonderful," I think. "I'll actually finish in time to meet my first office patient." I dislike the habitual lateness of doctors and fight a constant but losing battle against the clock. As I pass room 4, I notice Grace Maki sitting next to a frail shape lying motionless on the far bed. Grace is a nurse at the hospital, and we often work together in the emergency room. Today she is not in uniform and appears to be visiting a friend. I peek discreetly in and see that the patient is Mabel Sunderstrom. She's staring the other way and doesn't notice me. I nod to Grace and, feeling vaguely guilty for not stopping in, continue toward the nurses' station.

I don't recall ever actually meeting Mrs. Sunderstrom, although I have been peripherally involved with her case. Like many cancer patients, she has received almost all of her care in Duluth from one of their cancer specialists. Now that there is no further curative or even palliative treatment available, she has come home to die. Madeline Joswik, the county public health nurse, talked to me last week when I was on call and asked me to visit Mrs. Sunderstrom at her apartment to help with a problem. At that time, she wanted to stay home as long as she could to avoid the hospital. However, I didn't have time to visit her until evening, by which time Madeline had handled the problem herself and canceled the request. Apparently Mrs. Sunderstrom's condition worsened last night, and her husband felt he could no longer take care of her by himself. Dan Marks, one of my partners, admitted her to the hospital for supportive care, to make her

23

as comfortable as possible in the process of dying. She died within twenty-four hours.

Several days later, I am again at the nurses' station, finishing up. As I turn to leave, Grace Maki confronts me: "Why didn't you come in to see Mabel, David?" Grace is always straightforward, and it's not hard to tell she's upset.

For a second I'm confused. "You mean the other morning?" I say, as the memory of Grace sitting next to her friend returns along with that vague sense of guilt. "I don't know why....She wasn't my patient, I guess."

"She was dying, David. You could have helped her by at least talking with her. Why didn't you stop for just a moment?" Caught between anger and grief, she begins to cry.

A long-suppressed resentment rumbles inside me, and I suddenly don't care about Mrs. Sunderstrom or Grace's grief. "I can't take care of everybody, Grace. I can't respond to everybody's needs. She wasn't my patient, and there was no reason to stop in. Besides, it wouldn't have been just a moment. Those things take time!" I'm angry at her for dredging up my guilt, for confronting me, for making me late for supper again tonight.

"But she was such a beautiful person! You should have gotten to know her. You could have helped her."

"There are lots of beautiful people! I don't have the energy for every one of them." Grace is crying harder now. "I'm sorry for yelling, but I can't take care of everybody."

Grace's challenge stung me for some time. Looking back on the situation, I could hardly fault myself for not getting involved with a dying patient I neither knew nor had medical responsibility for. I reasoned that Grace was dealing more with her own grief (and perhaps guilt) than with any negligence on my part. It was a long time, however, before I understood why she provoked such an uncharacteristic outburst from me: she was saying out loud what I said to myself every time I failed to respond to someone's need.

Like many practicing physicians, I entered medicine out of a desire to be of service to people. Whatever other motives I may have had, my root ambition was to help, to respond to others' needs. What I failed to realize, however, was that the very nature of my work as a doctor would push me continually into the position of limiting the help I would give, of ignoring the needs of others. One of the pressing realities of my job was that I repeatedly found myself contradicting my own inner desire to be of service, a conflict that created in me a deep sense of guilt. It was this, I think, that erupted in response to Grace's anger and grief.

At the heart of this conflict lay the simple fact that there were too many patient needs for the time and energy I had available. When I found myself unable or unwilling to increase the time or energy I was investing in my work, those needs did not conveniently stop to allow me time to recover. It is, in fact, one of the basic dilemmas of the physician—to be caught between a desire to be of service and a need for respite. This conflict surfaced in many different ways throughout any given day, producing a long-term sense of alienation from my patients and encouraging me to deal with them as problems to be handled rather than as persons in need of care.

The appointment schedule, for instance, was a fundamental and necessary ingredient of my life. From my 8:00 A.M. arrival at the hospital until the 5:00 P.M. office closing hour, I was scheduled to see patients at definite intervals throughout the day. The purposes of such a schedule, of course, are to give each patient the amount of time his or her health problem requires, to reduce patient waiting, and to allow the physician to be efficient by providing an uninterrupted flow of patients—all legitimate functions. The receptionist would attempt to estimate the time each problem required and allocate that interval to the patient. Regardless of her success in estimating, the next patient would be there at the designated hour. (In our office we actually allowed more time for each visit than does the average family physician; thus, I usually saw twenty to twenty-five patients in each nine-to-five office day compared with the average thirty to thirty-five patients other family physicians might see.)

This scheduled appointment interval often was not enough for the patient's needs. What one patient thought to be a simple sore knee requiring only a few minutes could easily turn into a difficult diagnostic problem requiring a complete physical examination, drainage (through a large-bore needle) of some of the fluid from the knee, and laboratory testing to determine what kind of arthritis was present. After making an appointment, another patient would become aware of several other "little problems" and would have an entire agenda to cover with me during the ten or fifteen minutes we had available. Still another patient who complained of a headache would in fact be suffering from major personal and family emotional difficulties. Somewhere toward the end of the interview, as we were determining that the cause of the headache was not physical, he or she might say, "Well, I'm not surprised, Doc. I've been under a lot of stress lately." This could easily lead to an interview of thirty to forty-five minutes dealing with the real problem.

Each of these very understandable situations confronted me with a choice: either I could follow the patient's needs and stay with her until we had finished, or I could give her only the allotted appointment time and then terminate the interview, trying to reschedule for a later date. If I followed my inclination and stayed with the patient as long as was required, it meant that I fell behind schedule and would have to cut another patient short later in the day. If I tried to reschedule, it involved interrupting the patient, not responding to the underlying needs she might only be hinting at, hoping she would keep the rescheduled appointment time several days later, and finally charging for two appointments. Either way I found myself rushing to manipulate patients' needs into a "package" I could handle.

A similar situation arose regularly with emergency patients. As the only physicians in the county, we also staffed the hospital and the emergency room. We took turns being on call for the emergency room and being available to see patients who walked into the office without appointments. During the day we were on call, we were scheduled more lightly in the office to accommodate unscheduled needs. Since emergencies are unpredictable, however, we were frequently called to the emergency room during the middle of what was still a busy schedule. If the presenting problem was a true emergency, we would have to plunge in, respond to the situation, and return to the office an hour or more later to face an impossibly backed-up schedule. The only way to deal with such a crowded day was, of course, to deny patients complete service for the needs they presented: to shorten interviews, to perform briefer examinations, to ignore "secondary" problems not directly relevant to the chief complaint.

Frequently, the "emergency" patient did not have a true emergency, but was simply very worried about a particular problem and felt that it had to be taken care of immediately. During one busy afternoon, for instance, the emergency-room nurse calls the office to report that Arthur Desmond is in with a severe headache, stiff neck, and vomiting. Fearing meningitis, a stroke, or some other catastrophe, I quickly finish the office appointment and rush over to the hospital. The emergency room is darkened, and Arthur is lying on the cart with his eyes covered.

"What's the matter, Arthur?"

He takes the towel from his eyes and looks up at me. "Oh, hi, Doc. It's my head. It's killing me. Can you give me something to kill the pain?" I sit down beside the cart. "How long has it been bothering you, Arthur? When did it start?"

"Oh, it's been going on for a couple of months, Doc. We've been real busy down at the store, and I sometimes get these headaches real bad in the middle of the afternoon. I've been meaning to come up to the office to see one of you, but I couldn't find the time. Today Annie said she'd watch the store, so I called up to the office. They didn't have any appointments open, though, so I came over here."

"The nurse said you had a stiff neck and vomiting?"

"Well, not really vomiting, Doc, but I feel a little like throwing up when these headaches get bad. And I was out playing tennis with my boy day before yesterday, and my neck and shoulders are real stiff from that."

I continue my interview for a few minutes longer, and it becomes clear that Arthur does not have a true emergency. To evaluate his problem fully, however, will take at least half an hour. A thorough physical examination plus some laboratory tests will be necessary to make sure that this is a severe tension headache and not migraine, a brain tumor, or some rare cause of head pain. I am faced with the choice of completing my evaluation here, which will push me even further behind in my office schedule, or refusing to help Arthur now and rescheduling him for another day. A third alternative—evaluating him briefly, giving him some painkillers, and asking him to return to the office for a more complete evaluation—will probably result in his thinking he's already been taken care of and never following up on the complete evaluation, especially after he sees the emergency-room bill. It's a typical no-win situation for me as a physician. As usual, I stay with my "emergency" patient and complete the call, but not without resentment.

The effect of having a full schedule, additional patient problems, and emergency patients was to make me chronically late. It seemed to me that my days turned into a continual process of refusing complete service, shortening my time with patients, blunting my response to their problems.

Another ingredient in this needs-versus-time conflict was the internal pressure to be compulsively thorough in dealing with each patient problem. I had been trained as a physician to believe that disease in one part of the organism affects and is affected by the functioning of the rest of the body, so it was important to review the status of the patient's over-all health when dealing with almost any particular health problem. After ascertaining the nature of the patient's chief complaint, I was taught to inquire also about the eyes, ears, nose, and throat, to ask about the cardiovascular, respiratory, and gastrointestinal systems, to review sexual functioning, psychiatric well-being, social adjustment, and so on. I was regularly amazed at how a thorough "systems review" would turn up important new bits of information or even new problems more important to the patient's health than the presenting complaint. Thus, an encounter that began with the patient complaining of a persistent cough might easily develop into a lengthy discussion of smoking habits, a drinking problem, or job stress.

The obvious corollary is that almost every patient carries with her a set of major and minor problems of which she may not even be consciously aware. Physical problems abound, of course, but in our developed society the addictive problems of smoking, alcoholism, and obesity; the social problems of divorce, job dissatisfaction, child and spouse abuse, and social isolation; and the psychological problems of anxiety, depression, insomnia, and general boredom are quite literally everywhere. One does not need more than a modicum of interviewing skill to elicit discussion of many problems of immense importance, all discovered during the course of dealing with quite routine physical ailments.

Furthermore, as a physician I was defined by society, by the medical profession, and by my own expectations as the proper person—at least in our rural community—to handle all these problems. I was therefore under constant pressure to squeeze more service into shorter periods of time. When this pressure was combined with the roller-coaster pressures of the job, the emotional burden often seemed overwhelming. The blessing and the curse of medicine is that we physicians are privileged to share the most intense moments of life with our patients: birth, death, fear, sorrow, anxiety, disability, healing, joy. These moments are shared without the usual social barriers; thus, we are privy to the deepest of humanity's experiences. But with this privilege comes the burden of availability, of openness to the needs revealed at those intense times. Not surprisingly, I could not sustain the degree of openness required to go from deepest need to deepest need, and consequently I found myself refusing the very service that a major part of me was committed to giving.

I did not, of course, simply refuse to see patients or hear their complaints; rather, I withheld from them my complete attention. I neglected to ask about personal or social problems when performing the systems review. I asked directed questions calling for specific information about the nature of the patient's chief complaint rather than open-ended questions that might allow new problems to surface. Instead of sitting comfortably, I stood up during the interview, letting the patient know nonverbally that I was a busy man and she should stick to the "important" information. Merely by asking "Are there any other problems I can help you with?" I could subtly inform the patient that the interview was coming to a close. And if patients did not respond to my manipulations, I could be more direct: "Let me take care of this one problem first, and we'll get back to your other one another day." Most patients will not be consciously aware that they are being manipulated. But I knew I was denying my patients the totality of response they needed. I knew I was not providing that very availability I considered most important.

Perhaps even more emotionally burdensome, though, was my time on call. Since my partners and I were the only doctors in the county, we rotated call (a situation most rural physicians, who don't have three partners, would find pretty easy). At any time during that one-fourth of my life, I could be called for anything from a heart attack to a sore throat. Eating supper, visiting a friend, or deep in sleep, I had to be available immediately to patients. During that one-fourth of my life, I could not really relax or abandon myself to other concerns. During our slower winter season I didn't actually have to go to the hospital all that much. Nevertheless, the emotional drain of being on call came to feel like a subtle torture, slowly sapping my strength. During the summer, call was a rigorous, time-consuming necessity. The entire weekend, including most of the nights, frequently would be spent at the hospital, but I had to be ready to start work at eight o'clock Monday morning anyway.

Thursdays always seem the worst, perhaps because Friday is my day off and it's hard not to think of office closing time on Thursday as the beginning of my time off duty. Today, I finish with my last patient at 5:45 and begin on the list of phone calls that have accumulated during the day: two people who need prescriptions refilled, one who wants to know what the radiologist thought about her x-rays, and another who believes her husband is sick, though he refuses to come to the clinic. Could I call him at his office and find some excuse to make an appointment? Finally, there is old Mr. Kaikkonen, who calls me every three months to ask whether he needs to come in for a check on his high blood pressure. I tell him again that I would like to see him every three months and he needs only to call the receptionist to make an appointment. Once again, he seems surprised that it is so easy and promises to call the next morning.

The last note taped to my box informs me that two patients await me in the emergency room. The time on the note is 5:10. Marge must have taken the call just before she and the rest of the office staff left. My patients will have been waiting an hour. I call Marja, tell her not to expect me on time for supper, lock the clinic door, and walk over to the hospital. The hall outside the emergency room is filled with a dozen grimy campers and I begin to panic, but Grace Maki reassures me they are two parties of canoeists accompanying only two patients. The first young man, Tom Dorsey, twisted an ankle while portaging a canoe early this morning. It has taken them all day to paddle out of the wilderness and get into town. The ankle is swollen to perhaps twice its normal size. I examine it briefly and ask Grace to call Mark Todd in for an x-ray. I walk across the hall to our smaller, back-up emergency room to examine the second boy, who cut himself while cleaning fish. The laceration is small. It takes me only fifteen minutes to suture it and order a tetanus booster.

Even though I enjoy caring for these minor injuries, I'm tired and ready to be home with my family. I wait awhile in the doctors' lounge for Mark to finish with the x-rays. A stack of journals, which I always intend to read during these lulls, sits on the shelf but I can't summon the energy. I stare at the wall until Grace knocks on the door.

"It looks broken, David."

Mark and Grace have already diagnosed the obviously broken ankle on the young canoeist, but—according to strict protocol—I am the one to inform Tom. While he is still in the x-ray room, I show him the break on the films and explain that it will have to be casted. The bones are not badly displaced so there is no need to set the fracture, but the ankle is too swollen now for a cast. He will have to be in bed for a day or two with his ankle elevated before the swelling is down enough to allow for casting. I wheel Tom back to the emergency room and explain the entire situation again to the leader of the canoe trip. Do they want Tom to stay here in the hospital or should he go back home to Minneapolis? The group is on only the second day of their eight-day trip, so a complicated discussion ensues, including several long-distance phone calls to Tom's parents to check on insurance. While I wait for the group to make up its collective mind, I notice myself getting more and more impatient. I can't blame them for their difficulty in reaching a decision, but I want to get home. There are no other patients to attend to at the moment, so all I can do is stand around and wait for them. Half an hour later it is decided that Tom will stay here while the rest of the group continue on their trip. I do a brief physical exam and admit Tom to the hospital. I'll put on a cast Saturday or Sunday morning since I'm on call for the weekend.

I return to the doctors' lounge and begin changing clothes to go home when the nurse in charge of the hospital floor rings me on the telephone intercom. A Mr. Torrey is having an erratic heartbeat. My partner apparently admitted Mr. Torrey several days earlier with a mild and uncomplicated heart attack, but the nurses have noticed some dangerous-looking patterns on the heart monitor and they want me to evaluate the situation. I change back into my slacks and shirt, call Marja to give her a progress report, and walk out to the nurses' station.

Mr. Torrey's situation is not complicated, but since I am unfamiliar with his history, I have to review his entire chart, talk with him, and thoroughly evaluate his current tracings on the heart monitor as well as compare them with earlier tracings. It turns out that he has a long history of such erratic beats, and we needn't do anything to treat them, but it's taken me half an hour to reach that decision.

At eight-thirty I finally get back to the doctors' lounge and change into my running clothes. I make it a habit to run the two miles to and from work each day. It keeps me in shape and, perhaps more important, provides an emotional transition between work and home. Once I'm under way, some of the tension invariably dissipates. Arriving home, I towel off and sit down to the warmed-up food Marja has saved for me.

A sudden wave of tiredness engulfs me. Laurel, my oldest, begins to tell me about a book she's reading. Karin wants me to taste the first brownies she's ever baked. Kai, the youngest, just wants to play. Marja is tired after her day and wants a chance to sit down, too. But my energy is gone. I just can't seem to focus on the family around me. All I want to do is sit, eat my food, and stare at the newspaper. It never fails: If I get home after eight or eight-thirty, I just can't find the energy to relate to my family.

I finish dinner sullenly, read Kai a story, and put the girls to bed before sitting down to chat with Marja. But we talk for only five minutes before the phone rings: a young child in the emergency room with an earache. I drive down the hill and summon my remaining energy to appear both caring and reassuring. The entire round trip takes only thirty-five minutes, but it is already past my usual bedtime. As I pull into the driveway a little past eleven, I remember Margie Browning, a week overdue. I pray she doesn't go into labor tonight.

In addition to the official call schedule, I also found that people would present their needs to me at any time. Whether at home enjoying a book with my children, walking downtown to do some shopping, or sitting in church, I was always available for a brief consultation. (Someone once actually started asking about her mother's health before the closing hymn at church was over, and another patient literally tracked my partner to the trout stream where he was fishing on his day off.) I generally did not believe that people who asked for my opinion during these off-hours were being pushy or just looking for free advice. I hoped they saw in me the honest desire to be of service, not recognizing that their usually brief request was part of a much larger pattern that resulted in my feeling constantly besieged. As a part of this continuous unofficial call, I could be summoned at any time to deliver one of my obstetric patients or help a partner who needed assistance. Thus, I was never really off duty. Unless I physically left town, I had to be available to patient needs.

It is difficult to explain to a person who has not experienced the burden of being on call why it is so taxing. Call requires a degree of emotional readiness, of physical preparedness, that drained me as the years passed. After a weekend on call, I would be tired and feel desperate for rest even if I'd gotten all the sleep I needed and hadn't been very busy. If nothing else happened, being available was still work in itself.

I often found I was defending myself with subtle (and, I suppose, not so subtle) maneuvers. When patients asked me questions outside the office, I answered as briefly as possible after only a cursory description of the problem. I quickly referred people to the office, telling them I could not adequately answer without a longer interview and examination. I showed my discomfort so obviously that people felt guilty and would not ask again. To discourage questions on my days off, I would go downtown in only my scruffiest clothes ("Him, a doctor??!!") We took all our vacation time away from home, and even when I was officially on call, I would not infrequently find that in answering the telephone my highest priority was to avoid going down to the hospital (certainly not an attitude conducive to good medical care).

Health needs do not, of course, appear on schedule; and it did not in practice seem possible to educate people to call only the "on call" doctor for unscheduled problems, so the theoretical tidiness of a call schedule never seemed to work out. It is, of course, foolish to suppose that I could have responded to everyone's need. There seemed, however, to be no personally acceptable way of defining what the limits of my response should be. I would go through periods in which I felt I was constantly holding back; but then, filled with remorse, I would open myself to whoever presented themselves to me. This openness would last for days or weeks until its cumulative impossibility exhausted me. I seemed unable to find a middle way.

The feeling grew and grew that I had to protect myself from other people's needs, that they would tear me apart if I didn't take care of myself first. While my soul called for a life of service, my emotions called out for the life of a hermit.

Chapter 4

THE BOUNDARIES OF KNOWLEDGE

IT HAS BEEN a wonderfully normal pregnancy. Labor has gone smoothly, and now Donna and Jim Meeks are working together in the delivery room, a perfect picture of prepared childbirth. In a few moments their first child will enter the world here in our little hospital. The Meeks are from a small rural community fifty miles away. I am not their nearest doctor, but some years ago another couple from their area heard that I "believed in natural childbirth," and a small group of commuting patients began to see me for their obstetric care.

I have been flattered by their dedication and have tried to allow the couples as much control as possible over their own medical care. Jim accompanied Donna to most of the prenatal visits, and he has been extremely supportive during this labor. Donna has been pushing now for forty-five minutes, and the baby is about to be born. For me it has been a joy to be a part of the process.

"Dr. Hilfiker?…Fetal heart tones are up to 180!" Jean Appelton, the head nurse, is whispering to me, trying not to alarm Donna or Jim.

I look up at Donna, still pushing as hard as she can, at Jim straining right along with her. "Are you sure? Check it again!" This is the first sign of any complication—everything has been going so well. I'm not even sure what the elevation in the baby's heart rate might mean; usually a baby's heart rate slows with fetal distress.

Thirty seconds pass. Jean looks over at me. "Still 180."

The baby is so close to being born that there is not much time to consider intervening in the labor. "Donna, the baby's heart has speeded up a bit. I think it is important that we deliver it right away. Concentrate on pushing as much as you can." I make all the last-minute preparations for the delivery and ask the circulating nurse to unwrap the forceps in case Donna can't push the baby out quickly enough. But two contractions later, Donna pushes the baby's head through. Another few seconds and the rest of the body is born.

But the baby is limp, blue. I can detect a pulse of only 40 (instead of the normal 140), and the baby is not trying to breathe. My heart leaps into my throat. What's wrong? Even as I hurry to clamp and cut the umbilical cord so that I can bring the baby over to the emergency table, I notice how small it seems—less than five pounds. I was sure it was normal-sized.

We get the baby onto the table, under the infrared baby warmer. Celia, the anesthetist, and I begin resuscitation. Suctioning the mucus out of the throat, Celia inserts a tube into the trachea so she can breathe for the baby. I monitor the heart rate, which has dropped to 20, start external heart massage. Still no muscle tone, still blue. Jean pricks the baby's foot for a small blood sample to measure the blood sugar level: less than 40. So that's the trouble—hypoglycemia, or low blood sugar. But what's caused it? The baby's heart rate begins to rise, and I stop heart massage. The color improves. Finally the baby starts to breathe on its own, and we take the tube out of the trachea. But the baby is still floppy, with poor muscle tone. What do I do now? I know the baby needs sugar, but I'm not sure of the concentration, or how best to administer it.

I look over at Donna and Jim. They know, of course, that something is wrong. "Your baby's had some trouble getting started. Its heart rate was low, and it didn't start breathing right away. It seems a bit better now, but its still not moving normally. The blood sugar level's too low. I'm going to call the specialist in Duluth."

I'm grateful for the trust between us that allows this meager information to suffice for the moment. I check Donna quickly to make sure she's all right. Unfortunately, one of my partners is on vacation, and the other is at our satellite clinic thirty-five miles away, so I'll have to take care of both mother and baby simultaneously. I leave the delivery room for the nurses' station telephone.

Fortunately, the Newborn Intensive Care Unit in Duluth can get hold of the on-call newborn specialist for me immediately. I'm glad it's Mary Donaldson; she's always so reassuring. I describe the situation as succinctly as I can.

"Did you have a fetal monitor on during labor?" she asks. "What was the heart rate like then?"

"We don't have the monitor yet, Mary." How can I explain to her that our little hospital can't afford the $10,000 piece of equipment since it would be used only a few times a year? "The nurses listened, of course, but the heart rate seemed normal to them. We must have missed the decelerations in heartbeat."

"Yes, I think so. You said the baby's small? Did you get an ultrasound picture during pregnancy?"

"No, I didn't. The baby seemed normal size to me on examination, so I didn't get an ultrasound. I suppose I should have."

"Well, it might have tipped you off that something was wrong. But then, we don't always get them down here either, and these surprises can happen." She deliberates a minute. "Well, it seems the baby's probably small for gestational age; those babies often get severely hypoglycemic during labor. I think you should get some glucose in as soon as possible to prevent brain damage."

"OK," I say. "What route should we use for administration and what dosages?"

"I think an intraumbilical catheter would be best. Just give five percent glu—"

I interrupt her. "I've never put in an intraumbilical line." I feel so ignorant—one more skill, one more bit of information I should have. Putting a small plastic tube through the vein in the bellybutton shouldn't be difficult, but I've never done it before, and I know there can be complications. "I'm not even sure we have the correct supplies up here."

"Oh...well, then put an IV into a scalp vein and give a simple five percent glucose solution. If you can't get an IV going, you can put a gavage tube down into the baby's stomach and instill ten percent glucose; that would be better than nothing. These babies often have late complications too, so I'd suggest we come up in the ambulance and bring the baby down here for intensive care. It'll be much safer."

I review with Mary some of the details of the care we'll administer and the problems we might expect over the next several hours, and then return to the delivery room. The baby seems to have stabilized, but it is still floppy and blue. Fortunately Donna has only a small laceration of her vaginal opening, which I'll be able to repair easily when I've finished with the baby; she seems to be doing well otherwise. Jean and I work unsuccessfully for fifteen minutes trying to pass an IV catheter into one of the fragile veins of the baby's scalp. I haven't had to do this since my internship five years ago, and my skills have noticeably deteriorated. The small veins keep breaking. Finally we give up on the IV and put a tube into the baby's stomach. Fortunately, one of the newly recruited nurses on the staff used to work in a newborn intensive care unit. We get her out of bed (she had just finished the night shift), and she hurries in to help me manage the gavage tube, since I've never done that either. In the end, we succeed in instilling enough glucose to make the baby's blood sugar level rise to normal. I relax a little and turn my attention to Donna.

During the next two hours while we are waiting for the specialized neonatal transport ambulance from Duluth, the baby seems to do pretty well. I, however, am a nervous wreck! I remember vaguely that abnormal levels in blood minerals, trouble getting enough oxygen to the brain, and numerous other problems can plague babies who are small for their age, but I don't have the knowledge or skills, nor does our hospital have the equipment, to do the required testing or treatment. I keep wondering what's going to happen, what might go wrong. Finally, Mary arrives with the ambulance, an IV is started through the umbilicus, and the baby is transported to Duluth.

Over the next few days there are complications, and for a few months there is some concern about the possibility of cerebral palsy, but a year later Donna and Jim drive into my yard with their one-year-old baby boy. They have just been to Duluth, where Dr. Donaldson has pronounced the baby normal, and they want to share the good news with me. They express their gratitude for my care and my skills. I am deeply moved that they've come so far out of their way just to thank me; and also more than a little embarrassed by their praise, considering what I didn't know and couldn't do when their baby was born.

The explosion of medical knowledge that has taken place in recent decades has left all practicing physicians, but especially primary care physicians, in the eerie position of knowing that their skills and knowledge are too often incomplete for the task in which they are engaged. Medical science has expanded so rapidly, often completely reversing older concepts, that it is not humanly possible to keep abreast of developments even within specialties, much less in the whole of medicine. A nationally prominent cancer researcher gave a series of lectures to our medical school class. He told of returning to the meticulous notes he had taken while himself a medical student. "Ten years after I graduated," he said, "they were all lies! Things had changed so drastically that I couldn't trust any of my notes for accurate information." Though exaggerated, his observation is essentially accurate. Basic concepts, to say nothing of skills and procedures, are developing so rapidly that it is impossible to stay current with it all.

My immediate response, of course; was to do everything I could to keep up. I read two weekly medical journals and thumbed through several others for new developments. I attended approximately one hundred hours per year of continuing medical education courses. Our small group of doctors met regularly in a "journal club" to review with each other new things we had read or heard about. On two separate occasions I took four to six weeks of further training in a residency program. I consulted frequently by phone with the specialists in Duluth to whom I referred my difficult cases. I carefully read the consultations returned to me in the mail, looking for new approaches to problems. Despite all these efforts, I felt like a child trying to protect his sand castle from the inexorable onrush of the tide.

My second approach to the problem was to try to limit my practice. "As long as you know what it is that you don't know," I told myself, "and limit yourself to the things you do know, then you won't get into trouble." So I referred more and more patients to specialists. I tried to pick out the women who were going to have problems during labor, whose babies were too small. I sent to Duluth some of the trauma patients I probably could have handled. My phone calls to my specialist friends in Duluth became ever more frequent (four or five separate calls a day would not have been unusual), and I arranged for them to see the patients about whom I had doubts.

Even so, there were unforeseen problems. Patients would suddenly appear—quite literally in the case of Donna's baby—demanding intensive care I was not equipped to give. Cardiac patients would be in too precarious a state during the first hours after their heart attacks for transfer, so we had to develop a full-scale coronary care unit in our hospital and attend those patients as best we could. Even routine problems could suddenly turn out to be much more complex than originally anticipated.

In the end, it is really not possible to "know what it is that you don't know." Medicine is always uncertain. Referring to specialists everyone about whom I had doubts would have meant treating very few patients on my own. Further, if I restricted my care only to the simplest problems, those skills I did possess would atrophy, and I would be even less able to deal with patients' illnesses.

The final compromise, though perhaps not theoretically satisfying, allowed me at least to continue practicing. Telling myself that I was adequately handling a high percentage of the patient problems presented to me, I tried to convince myself that my limitations in knowledge and skill were not so important as I might think. Thus, I continued to do my best, combining my attempts to keep up with the knowledge explosion with my attempts to limit myself and utilize consultants.

But nothing could obscure my frequent collisions with my own deficiencies in knowledge and skill. Despite my best efforts, I failed to make certain diagnoses, performed procedures incorrectly, neglected to refer for proper treatment—all for lack of proper knowledge. The contradiction remained: I was forced into diagnosis and treatment recognizing that, in one sense, I could never be adequately qualified. Sometimes it seemed that the concept of family practice was unsound; perhaps all my patients should be attended by specialists, whose knowledge in their particular field would at least be more complete than mine. But I knew there were other difficulties when patients were attended exclusively by specialists. Complaints outside a particular physician's specialty tended to be ignored. Problems like alcoholism, depression, or family stress could not easily be diagnosed or treated by a specialist who saw the patient only occasionally. Patients with vague complaints were shunted from one doctor to another as first the cardiologist, then the lung specialist, and finally the neurologist determined that the chest pain was not caused by the organs for which they were responsible. Specialist care tended to be very expensive, as each physician performed her own separate history and physical evaluation and then ordered her own battery of particular tests that she felt necessary to proper care. In my case, since specialists were 110 miles away, I knew my patients could not rely on them exclusively for their care. So there seemed to be no option except continuing to work in the face of my ignorance.

While the information explosion in the medical sciences left me feeling continually benighted, I was also overwhelmed by the ever-present need for what our behavioral science professors had blandly called "interpersonal skills" with which I was to respond to the "psycho-social needs" of my patients. In real life this meant figuring out how to cajole Jane Michaels into believing that her headaches were the result of her life-style, not of a brain tumor. Jane saw me frequently for a variety of medical problems. At forty she was severely overweight, smoked heavily, had high blood pressure, lived in a disastrous marriage, and had major difficulties with her children.

"Dr. Hilfiker, you have to do something. These headaches are killing me. My husband gets mad when I have them, and I can't do nothing with the kids. All I can do is lay in bed and sleep. My head hurts so bad if I try to get up. You told me last time they came from the trouble Dick and I was having, but we're getting along OK now, and these headaches are worse than ever. I read in a magazine that brain tumors can cause headaches, and I don't want no brain tumor. You gotta do something."

Eight months ago Jane saw me for her headaches, as she had done a year ago and two years before that. I have evaluated her twice before with some thoroughness, and in my own mind I am convinced her headaches are due to the stress of a most difficult life. She hasn't stayed with the counselor I recommended, however, and I have no ready cures for most of her social problems. Today, I ask her some questions about the headaches to make sure there is nothing new or suspicious, and I examine her briefly to rule out any serious disease. "Jane, you don't have a brain tumor," I tell her after my examination. "I still think these headaches are from all the stress you're under. Why don't—"

"Dr. Hilfiker, why do you always talk to me about stress! That magazine says doctors can't tell if there's a brain tumor without getting that special new x-ray of the head, cat scam or something. How do you know I'm not really sick? You just ask me some questions and look in my eyes. I want to get that x-ray to make sure there's no brain tumor."

"Jane, that x-ray costs a lot of money; besides, your symptoms don't warrant—"

"Dr. Hilfiker, I want that x-ray. You're treating me like this 'cause I'm on welfare. I read about that, too. If you won't help me, then I'll have to find a doctor who will. You always think everything's just mental. I thought you was supposed to help people!" Putting on her coat, Jane stalks out of the examining room.

Jane will probably call back in a day or two to apologize. We've been through this before. But I realize I do not have the skills to reach Jane and offer her help. I can tell her she doesn't have a physical illness, but my ability to move from there into the areas where Jane really needs help is very limited.

Jane's was not an atypical situation. A high percentage of patients (some studies indicate more than half) coming to primary care physicians will have no demonstrable organic disease and will respond poorly or not at all to purely medical attempts to alleviate their symptoms. Even those patients whose disease has an obvious physical cause will frequently suffer emotional distress or exhibit actual psychiatric symptoms in combination with their organic illness. To complicate matters further, physicians must contend with small numbers of problem patients—the "clingers," the "demanders," the "help-rejecters," the "deniers."[5] We must possess special techniques both to take care of these patients and to understand the complicated feelings they stir up in us.

Even the routine health consumer today expects the physician not only to provide accurate diagnosis and treatment for organic illness, but also to alleviate symptoms, provide sympathy and support, and relieve the fear associated with illness. Furthermore, physicians are working with intensely emotional aspects of life—suffering, fear, sexuality, and death.[6] The vast emotional and spiritual needs of patients, ranging from the terminally ill cancer patient to the embarrassed adolescent wondering about venereal disease, require of the physician specific skills and a high level of maturity. One must be able to elicit information without embarrassing, communicate a diagnosis without aggravating fear, reassure without falsely comforting, and prescribe treatment without oversimplifying the problem or the expected outcome. Even such a simple matter as providing effective reassurance to a worried patient is a specific skill that has to be learned;[7] and these were not patient needs that I could refer to a counselor or psychiatrist, for they are an integral part of daily practice.

Owen Baker brings his sixteen-year-old son Roger into the office, demanding that I do a test to see whether Roger had been smoking marijuana the night before. Despite the fact that such tests are not routinely available, it probably would be possible to comply with his demand. But I'm bothered by the situation. What's wrong with the relationship between Owen and his son that he'd even consider dragging him in here for a urine test? What will be the ultimate effect on their relationship of forcing Roger to take such a test? Do Owen's concern and his way of expressing it have anything to do with his own alcoholism, which he refuses to acknowledge? Would it be possible to involve them in some kind of family counseling without violating Roger's privacy by forcing him to take the test? And how can I refer them anywhere when Owen is so unready to acknowledge his need for counseling? As I trip clumsily through this emotional minefield with Owen and his son, I realize how poorly prepared I am to help them deal with these issues. Interviewing Roger alone, I find him to be a bright and articulate young man who maintains without defensiveness that he hasn't ever used marijuana—although he thinks he might try it eventually. He is angry about the scene his father has created but is not opposed to the urine test. Asking Owen to join us, I tell him I think I can arrange the test, but that it will probably be expensive. He abruptly starts talking about all the drugs he thinks are being used at school, and eventually leaves the office without ordering the test. As is often the case, I wonder whether or not I have blundered through once again without doing any great damage to anyone.

Why hadn't I been better prepared for this in medical school? I think back to the years of lectures in which the emphasis was so heavily on understanding the workings of the body in health and disease. The diagnosis was everything! Understanding which organ had failed, how it had failed, and what the prognosis was: that was the point of those lectures. Even in our clinical training, when we were actually seeing patients and following them in the hospital, the emphasis remained on diagnosis and to some extent on medical treatment. We were so busy trying to figure out what was wrong and what should be done that there was no time or energy left to understand how an acute medical problem fit into the life of the patient. We were so overwhelmed by the problems of diagnosis and treatment that a patient's inability or unwillingness to participate in our suggested treatment seemed too much to worry about. Even those few professors who tried to teach us "behavioral sciences" could not keep our attention; it all seemed so vague and irrelevant compared with the pathophysiology of diabetes.

The assumption in medical school seemed to be that our general common sense would take care of us when it came time to use our interpersonal skills. I suppose our professors were just as uncomfortable as I am in dealing with the realities of patients who don't trust us, of families who have deserted the obnoxious patient, of patients who never seem satisfied with the explanations we offer. Perhaps our professors never taught us because they didn't really know themselves. Everybody was more comfortable dealing with the "hard" sciences of pathology and neuroanatomy. It came as quite a shock, once I was out in practice, to discover that my common sense was not developed enough to help my patients through the chaos of their emotional response to illness.

Not only are physicians expected to have complete knowledge of the technical aspects of medicine and a well-developed ability to communicate; our society, I soon learned, also expects its doctors to be expert in virtually everything that has to do with human well-being. The physician's supposed expertise in dealing with severe psychiatric disturbances (traditionally a very weak area for most doctors anyway) has in recent years been broadened to include all emotional disturbances. The physician should be an expert in marriage counseling, sex therapy, drug and alcohol abuse intervention and treatment. She should be able to treat the problems of aging, loneliness, anxiety, adolescent crises, and child abuse.

The physician's expertise in matters of disease has been expanded to make her an expert in health as well. She should be able to help patients lose weight, stop smoking, start exercising, change their diets, have a more fulfilling sex life, and rear their children properly. The fact that there are separate bodies of knowledge and specialists in each one of these areas is ignored. And medical professionals have allowed themselves to accept these expectations. Today practitioners can go to continuing-education courses in any of these areas and come home with a modicum of expertise. There are, of course, individual physicians who have become truly competent in one or another of these areas. One of my former partners became interested in marriage problems, began doing marriage counseling, attended continuing-education courses, read the relevant journals, and after several years became greatly skilled in that area. But his skill grew out of his special interest, extra training, and experience. His training as a physician did not automatically endow him. Nevertheless, we doctors expect ourselves to be competent in each of these areas; and so I would regularly find myself confronting an alcoholic about his drinking, realizing for the hundredth time that I was never trained for anything like this situation. I would notice myself offering the couple with marriage problems only vague platitudes rather than skilled, specific counseling. I would expect myself to guide a person through a weight-loss program, yet have no idea where to start.

Early in my career I was heady with the prestige and power that came from the feeling that I would be able to fulfill everyone's expectations. Ingrid Karhonen began seeing me for a number of physical complaints. After examining her at separate successive appointments for headache, heart palpitations, insomnia, and stomach pains, I finally suggested that there might be some underlying emotional stress causing her ever-changing symptoms, and I recommended that we spend some time in counseling trying to get at the root of her problems. She was remarkably receptive to my idea, and I confidently set up our first appointment.

Our initial hour together went smoothly. I am a good listener, and I was able to encourage her to talk about a multitude of emotional problems. At age twenty-five with four young children, Ingrid was feeling swamped by the responsibilities of being a mother. She and her husband had recently moved to our community, and she was feeling lonely and isolated. She was resentful of her husband, whose independent logging business kept him away from home for long periods of time and who was not inclined to help much with the housework or parenting; Matt was also much older than Ingrid, a Finnish immigrant without much patience for his wife's physical symptoms. During the second hour, Ingrid continued to talk as I encouraged her to ventilate her feelings. She had come from a broken home and had a poor relationship with a domineering mother who still tried to run her daughter's life long-distance from San Francisco. Her brothers and sisters frequently came for visits and ended up crowding Ingrid's small house and straining her limited food budget for several weeks at a time; Ingrid was unable to ask them to leave. Her oldest boy, Stevie, was becoming a severe discipline problem in the fourth grade. By our third appointment, I was beginning to get the picture: Ingrid was an emotionally weak person, dominated by her husband, mother, siblings, and children, and unable to exert control over her life. It became very clear to me why she was having so many physical problems: there was no acceptable way for her to express her feelings, so they remained bottled up inside, finally manifesting themselves as headaches, palpitations, insomnia, and stomach aches.

In the succeeding interviews, Ingrid kept talking about her many problems. I was still a good listener, but I found myself absolutely unable to get Ingrid to do anything except complain about her life. I knew we were at what my behavioral-science professors would have called a "therapeutic impasse." I knew that there were several possible ways around our dilemma, things a therapist might do to encourage Ingrid to understand her behavior. But I was absolutely unable to maneuver us around the impasse. We talked on and on for many weeks, but there was no movement at all. Finally, Ingrid stopped coming, and I didn't call to encourage her to return. Our experiment had fizzled. Several months later Ingrid came in to see one of my partners, complaining of severe headaches.

While I knew I was supposed to respond to the needs of the "whole person," that there was more to headaches than brain tumors, I had also learned that good intentions can carry one only so far. I knew I was a sensitive, caring person who was very willing to listen. I knew I was a "good doctor." Feedback from colleagues and patients was positive. But I recognized that in a wide variety of areas I was continually getting in over my head. My response to this situation was insecurity and self-doubt. I suspect other physicians may respond to similar stresses by becoming excessively compulsive or overly authoritarian, but the situation itself cannot be avoided. As physicians we are constantly confronting our own ignorance.

Chapter 5

UNCERTAINTY

"I'VE BEEN SICK FOR the past six weeks, David. It started gradually with some sweats and chills and then got worse. I've felt weak and tired. I've got no appetite. I've lain in bed for a week now, but it hasn't seemed to help. What's going on?"

Carl Fitch is a close friend about my own age. I know him well enough to be sure that he wouldn't have come to the office unless he felt really sick. I can tell he's worried, but as I interview him and examine him I find nothing specific to explain his symptoms. I'm worried, too. Six weeks is a long time to be sick; his symptoms may represent a more serious underlying illness.

Fortunately, Carl has comprehensive medical insurance allowing us to investigate his illness without much regard to cost. I send him over to the hospital laboratory for an initial series of tests, but when he returns several days later for a consultation, none of the tests points definitively to an answer.

"Well, Carl, our initial lab tests look pretty normal. I'm not sure what's going on. The fact that your examination so far looks normal puts serious physical illness further down on the list of my concerns. You may have a persistent virus troubling you. Some of your white cells look a little reactive, suggesting a lingering infection, but I can't be sure. How about emotional stresses?"

Carl counsels people as part of his job, too, and he has observed how emotional tension can lead to physical symptoms. We discuss the pressures he is under, which, as for everybody else these days, are considerable. We talk about his family, his marriage, career satisfaction. There is stress, to be sure, but nothing has changed drastically in the last six months. There is no obvious diagnosis in this area, either. "Well, we're pretty much back where we started," I tell him. "It's very likely a persistent virus, but it also could be emotional exhaustion, and I can't completely rule out serious underlying illness, either."

"So...what do I do?" he asks. "I'm worried about the serious illness. How likely is it? I feel pretty sick."

"I'd like to be able to give you a percentage, Carl, but I can't. I'd guess that the chance of something serious is quite small, maybe one or two percent, but I don't know for sure. Why don't you take another week off from work and stay in bed? Let's see if that will help."

Carl remains quite concerned, and my doubts are not resolved either, so we decide to do some further tests while he is resting. When he returns a week later, he still feels the same and his tests still suggest an undetermined viral illness. Since I can't be sure, however, I think through the more exotic diseases: a smoldering infection of the heart valves, fungal infection of the lungs, hidden leukemia, Hodgkin's disease; the list goes on and on. Carl and I decide to search more thoroughly for evidence of serious underlying illness. Over the next week I order perhaps $1,000 worth of laboratory studies in addition to giving him another complete physical exam.

By the end of the third week since our initial interview, Carl is beginning to feel somewhat better. Most of his tests have returned with normal results, but there are still some virus studies which will not come back for several weeks. I do my best to reassure my friend. "I think it's a virus, Carl. You're getting better. Your tests are normal. Why don't we just wait and watch. Continue to rest and take care of yourself, let me know if anything new develops, and we'll let time give us the answer."

"Well, OK. I guess there isn't anything else to do. But are you sure there isn't anything serious going on? I've never felt this way for such a long time before...."

I almost consider lying, just to be reassuring, but decide to remain honest with him. "No, I can't be sure you don't have some bizarre illness just starting up. I don't think so, but I can't be sure."

After several more weeks, Carl does recover, and we do get some evidence suggestive of a viral infection. But we never make a firm diagnosis. Throughout Carl's illness both of us have lived with the discomfort of lingering doubt.

Medicine is a highly uncertain science. Not only is there far too much knowledge required for one person to grasp it all; but, even at its best, medicine usually cannot provide the definitive answers that patients and practitioners alike would want. Dr. J.D. McCue has written:

> Much of medical training consists of learning to cope with pervasive
> uncertainty and with the limits of medical knowledge. Making
> serious clinical decisions on the basis of conflicting, incomplete, and
> untimely data is routine....The physician is palpably relieved to
> encounter a typical presentation of a definable illness—for once the
> stress of gambling without knowing the odds (or often even the
> game) is avoided.[8]

Although there are obvious exceptions (lacerations, broken bones, earaches,
bladder infections, to name a few), the majority of illnesses that patients
bring their doctors are difficult or impossible to diagnose with any certainty,
and their treatment is equally problematic. The everyday complaints of
colds, viruses, skin rashes, bellyaches, fevers, childhood fussiness,
sleeplessness, coughs, and indigestion are usually of uncertain etiology. The
physician can often provide useful information and support to the patient
("It doesn't seem serious," "It will pass on its own," or "It's normal to
experience this"), but he usually cannot offer a precise diagnosis nor be sure
he is helping in the cure. More serious problems of chronic disease
(arthritis, heart disease, diabetes, cancer) usually are easier to diagnose
(although the precise nature and cause of these conditions are often elusive),
but even here the physician can rarely offer a cure or provide a certain
prognosis.

Unfortunately, it is highly stressful for patient and physician alike to live
with uncertainty. When I was a student and an intern, I would marvel at an
often-repeated process. After a careful interview, meticulous examination,
and thorough laboratory evaluation, no definitive diagnosis of a patient
would seem apparent. At that point, the supervising physician often simply
declared that, in his opinion, the patient suffered from the "X" problem. X
usually would turn out to be a diagnosis such as "psychosomatic
complaints," "such-and-such virus," or some obscure disease, all of which
diagnoses were incapable of proof or disproof. We students and interns
would murmur approvingly at the physician's wisdom (mostly because we
couldn't think of anything else to offer), and we would all pass on to the
next patient.

It was not until I had been in practice for several years that I realized the
largely unconscious dynamic behind that familiar phenomenon. The doctor
knew his students expected him to be able to make a secure diagnosis.
When he could not do this, he needed something to protect his image of

himself. So he had his own list of "wastebasket diagnoses" into which he threw all the problems that seemed to fit nowhere else. The stress of his own expectations and those of others in the face of endemic uncertainty tempts the physician to deny the complexities and limitations of medicine.

Not only is such uncertainty anxiety-producing for all concerned, it also subtly changes the nature of medical practice. Since neither definite diagnosis nor positive cure can be provided in most patient encounters, the physician must limit himself to doing as much as possible to rule out serious disease, prevent serious complications, provide information about the expected course of the problem, and offer, if possible, some alleviation of the patient's symptoms—an endeavor that combines science and art in a complex set of maneuvers through the murky waters of uncertainty. Unfortunately, this process may fulfill the expectations of neither patient nor physician.

Consider the following brief appointment: I enter the examining room to find Adele Johnson sitting uncomfortably on the table. I know her slightly since we have daughters in the same class in school. Thirty-one years old, the mother of three young children, a part-time employee at a small office downtown, Adele looks and sounds terrible—bloodshot eyes, runny nose, a hoarse voice.

"I've had this cold and sore throat for a week, Doc, and I can't seem to shake it. I'm weak and chilled, and I feel awful. I can hardly get through the morning at the office, much less the rest of the day. Terry is starting to come down with it, too, and I don't want the rest of the kids to get it. Can you give me something to knock it out?"

I avoid her questions and ask when the first symptoms started and what else has been bothering her. I ask briefly about other organ systems in the body. Although I expect from the moment I walk in that she has a cold, a "viral upper respiratory infection," my first concern is to make sure that there is nothing else going on. I examine her respiratory tract carefully, looking for other problems: no sign of ear infection, no evidence of an abscess near her tonsils, lungs clear without pneumonia. Adele seems impatient with all my fussing. "It's just a cold, Doc. All I want is a shot or something to get rid of it. We're supposed to go away this weekend and I have to get better."

When I've finished my questions and examination, I sit down on my stool. Adele is still perched on the examining table, wrapped in her sheet. "Well, I think you're right, Adele. It appears to be just a cold, but your throat looks pretty raw. I'd suggest doing a throat culture to make sure that you don't have strep throat."

She looks at me impatiently. "Is that going to help me get better? I heard they cost fifteen bucks."

"No, it won't help you get better at all, Adele." I think to myself that there must be some way to tape this conversation so I don't have to repeat it three times a day for the next twenty years. "But the only way to know for sure whether or not you have strep throat is to do a culture. I can't tell just by looking. If it is strep, you'll need penicillin to prevent the possibility of your getting rheumatic heart fever later on."

"Well, why don't you just give me the penicillin right now and knock the thing out without a culture? That's all I really want, Doc, is to get rid of this thing." I can feel her frustration rising.

"Penicillin won't do a thing for you if this is a virus, and there are dangers in using antibiotics needlessly. Even if it is strep, the penicillin won't get you better any faster. The only reason I'd recommend it would be to prevent the small chance of getting rheumatic heart fever that can follow a strep throat."

Adele looks down on me in disbelief. "You mean you won't give me anything to make me feel better? Doc, we've got to go away this weekend. It's really important!"

In a small corner of my mind, I am amused at Adele's implication that if she can just convince me of the importance of her getting well, I will reach deep into my magic black bag and pull out a special medicine I reserve only for times when it is "really important."

"Well, I can suggest some things that will make you feel better. Aspirin, gargling, hot liquids, and throat lozenges will all help your throat feel better, but I think the most important thing to do is to go to bed. You can't push yourself with a job, kids, and a household and expect to get well. Take a few days off and just lie around."

"I can't do that, Doc. There's too much to do before the weekend. Why don't you just give me some of that penicillin, and we'll forget about the culture. Penicillin's always worked before."

We spar for a few minutes more. When it's all over, Adele gets her penicillin shot without the culture, a reasonable compromise medically. The compassionate part of me hopes that the placebo effect of the shot will help her feel better, but a more self-righteous part of me hopes her virus will linger a few more days to prove that I was right about the penicillin.

Adele's main concern, of course, was getting better. Although I too hoped she would get better soon, I knew that I couldn't do much to speed that process except encourage good health habits that Adele already knew about but was ignoring. My main concerns were making a rough diagnosis, ruling out any serious illnesses, checking for strep in order to prevent the small chance of rheumatic fever, and then making some suggestions about how she could manage herself during the course of her illness. Thus, we were coming to our appointment with different priorities. It's little wonder that both of us felt frustrated.

The physician is a clinician who must make decisions on the basis of probabilities. Most patients, however, have little experience with this method of decision-making and are often unwilling to accept the uncertainty of medicine. If I express doubt that a particular diagnosis or treatment is completely reliable, this doubt may seem to my patient to be evidence that I am not competent, or haven't been thorough, or don't care. In Carl Fitch's case, for instance, I could tell him that the probability of serious disease was quite low, but I could not honestly tell him not to worry about it. Almost all decisions in medicine are made (whether consciously or not) on the basis of probabilities. When I am quite explicit about this process, it can become—even with sophisticated patients—a time-consuming matter (and the pressures of my schedule, if nothing else, often made me want to pull back from such explanations).

Terry Adolphson, for instance, was a thirty-six-year-old friend with a terrible family history of heart disease: all the male family members on his father's side had died with heart attacks before the age of forty. Terry had recently developed pain in the chest, or angina, suggesting that he too had a serious disease of the coronary arteries, the small blood vessels leading to the heart, a disease that could progress to a heart attack and quite possibly death. Recent articles in the medical literature had suggested that certain patients with angina not only had better pain relief but also lived longer if they underwent coronary-artery bypass surgery than if they were treated only with medicines. On the other hand, these patients had a definite chance of dying during surgery.

To complicate matters further, even the process of examining Terry to discover whether he had disease in the arteries which should be operated upon required a special examination of the coronary arteries (coronary arteriography). There was a small (usually less than one percent) chance of heart attack and even death during such an examination.

As I discussed the situation with Terry, I realized that in order to recommend this single test, I had to review with him some very complicated medical studies. There were, at that time, differences of opinion among leading cardiologists about who should receive coronary bypass surgery, since the studies had not yet shown convincingly that such surgery was advantageous. Two studies of which I was aware had followed for five years patients who had symptomatic and arteriographically proven heart disease. In each study, the patients were randomly divided into two groups. One group had surgery, and the other was treated only with medicine. The studies showed that for blockages in certain coronary arteries there was no real difference in survival between the surgical and nonsurgical groups; in some cases the nonsurgical group even did better. However, for blockages in other coronary arteries—the left main artery, for example—a greater number of patients were alive five years later in the subgroup that chose surgery than in the subgroup that was treated with medicine alone.

Terry and I reviewed the reasons for his undergoing the coronary arteriography and the chances of his dying during the examination. Since there was no reason even to consider the arteriography test unless he was interested in surgery, we went over the studies that seemed to show advantage for the surgical treatment of some patients. We examined what the literature had to say about the statistical chances of dying during the surgery, as well as the chances of surviving with or without surgery. I realized that I was not merely informing Terry about a complex disease involving complex therapy but also about a method of decision-making which, though routine in medical circles, was quite alien to him. Medical science could only report what had happened to groups of other people; these statistical "certainties" could not be translated into an individual certainty—into a reliable prediction for Terry. The discussion was time-consuming and therefore expensive. It took him several days just to absorb the concepts. My only alternative (on the surface, the easier path) would have been to ignore this reasoning process and tell him: "I, as your physician and your friend, recommend that you have this operation. Trust me." But the situation was not at all black and white. It involved not only uncertainties but values. Did Terry wish to take a chance on death resulting from an "unnatural" surgical intervention or on "natural" death as a result of avoiding surgery? Did he wish to risk a smaller chance of dying sooner (with the surgery) or a larger chance of dying in the indefinite future? Although I could interpret the medical information for Terry so that he could understand it, ultimately he had to take responsibility for the decision.

Even so, I did not share with Terry certain more complex uncertainties. I decided not to complicate the discussion further by reminding Terry of the uncertain nature of any statistical analysis. Perhaps even the studies that showed improvement after surgery were the result of coincidence or of some unknown difference between the surgical and nonsurgical groups. A statistical analysis of the studies could tell me there was only a five-percent chance that the results were due to coincidence, but we could not be 100 percent sure even that the studies were reliable. Nothing seems 100 percent certain in medicine! But Terry had enough uncertainty in his life. I chose to keep my "five percent probabilities" to myself.

Terry decided, after much thought and consultation, to proceed with the coronary arteriography; and it indeed showed a blockage in those coronary arteries which, the statistics indicated, it would be advantageous to bypass. He underwent the surgery, but the first nine months after the operation were difficult. Symptoms continued, a repeat coronary arteriogram was required, and there was much uncertainty about the wisdom of surgery. Had I initially talked Terry into the surgery by insisting that he trust me, that trust would have been severely threatened by all the unforeseen complications he experienced. Instead, he was able to face his future with some equanimity because he had made a reasonable decision based on adequate, if sometimes frustrating, information.

This statistical basis for decision-making permeates day-to-day medical practice, although not usually as dramatically as in Terry's situation. Because of the time-consuming nature of the discussion, we physicians often are tempted to leave out the description of the process when talking with patients, thus leaving them with the impression that there is much more certainty than actually exists. The ensuing confusion when the outcome is poor frequently leaves the patient feeling angry and betrayed, sure that the physician was guilty of some gross negligence. For his part, the physician is impatient and angry with the patient's "unrealistic" expectations and, not infrequently, guilt-ridden for not fulfilling them.

Many patients acquire knowledge about illness through simplified information in newspapers and magazine articles, through their own friends' experiences, or even through overwrought hospital melodramas on television in which dramatic cures are regularly performed. Thus, they tend not to understand the necessity to work with probabilities. Patients and physicians, then, are poorly prepared to communicate with each other about the uncertainties of a patient's particular problem.

Mort Jesperson is a forty-seven-year-old plumber forced into early retirement by multiple sclerosis, a tragic neurological disease in which the nerves gradually deteriorate, leaving the patient with weakness, loss of sensation, severe tingling, and a multitude of other difficult problems. As an added frustration, multiple sclerosis is a disease of exacerbations and remissions: that is, it gets worse and then better and then worse again, all with no apparent reason. The usual course of the disease is a gradual decline, but the patient can frequently improve for months at a time, only to regress suddenly to a point even worse than before. This characteristic leads to hundreds of newfound "treatments": anything that happened to a patient just prior to the spontaneous improvement can be seen as a miraculous new cure. Since the disease also has no satisfactory medical treatment, the lay press is full of remedies—some crazy, some reasonable. Medical science itself has a very difficult time evaluating the treatments. Sophisticated studies are needed to be sure that a placebo effect is not responsible for the "cure," since it is well known that a patient's belief that she will improve frequently results in sustained remissions of the disease. Consequently, even the medical press is full of case reports of success in the treatment of multiple sclerosis.

Mort had increasingly severe disease over the years I was his physician. Every six months or so his wife would bring him into the office for evaluation, and he frequently showed me literature about a new treatment, which he would ask me to evaluate. At first, he wanted me to hospitalize him for intravenous doses of a powerful drug. This treatment had once been popular among physicians, but recent reports had been disappointing. I tried to explain this to Mort, but he was so sure the drug had helped him during previous treatments that I finally agreed to supervise its administration. At the next visit, he wanted to know about megavitamin therapy and then about some herbs he had read about in a magazine for multiple-sclerosis patients. During my first years working with Mort, I was impatient. Why couldn't he understand how difficult it was to evaluate these treatments properly? Why did he keep trying to talk me into giving him what I considered dangerous treatments with little hope of success? Why didn't he catch on as, year after year, each new treatment was ultimately discredited? As time went by and I continued to listen to Mort, I began to see his side of things. He had an incurable disease that was ravaging his life with little or no future to look forward to. He was not interested in how small the probabilities were or in the potential dangers. For him, any chance of even temporary improvement was important, a goal worth the risk. He saw me, I'm sure, as a stiff young know-it-all, continually squelching his hopes for a few days of relief. Mort and I were meeting each other from two different worlds. It took a great deal of patience on both our parts to continue our relationship.

Other patients were less understanding than Mort. Adele Johnson, for instance, did not really care about my opinion that penicillin would not help her viral upper respiratory infection. I could have quoted her chapter and verse of scientific studies demonstrating that "within 95 percent confidence limits," penicillin was no more effective than placebos. She "knew" that penicillin helped: "Everybody knows that. Two years ago I was sick for two months with some virus and I finally managed to talk the doctor into some penicillin. I was better in a week." The lengths to which the medical profession had to go to discredit Laetrile is recent evidence that physicians and patients simply perceive this aspect of health and disease differently.

The extremely unfortunate result of the inherent uncertainty of medicine and of the methods of coping with that uncertainty is that the patient has expectations of the physician which the physician cannot possibly fulfill—a discrepancy that leads easily to dissatisfaction and distrust. So stressful is the uncertainty itself and so difficult is it to communicate fully with the patient that the physician is tempted to avoid explanations altogether. It seems easier to retreat behind a mask of stony indifference, to appear certain, to reassure the patient that the doctor knows what is best. For her part, the patient cannot understand why the doctor seems so evasive, why he won't say what he is thinking, why so many questions are left unanswered. Because the fundamental issue of the uncertainty of medicine has not been addressed, both physician and patient are left feeling misunderstood.

In my own practice, I came to dread the simple complaints such as colds, viruses, and headaches, not so much because I was worried that I was missing something serious, but because people seemed so disappointed with the indefinite results of my examination and treatment. Often I would "know" (with a high degree of probability) before I stepped into the examining room that the next patient had a viral upper respiratory infection, and that I was not going to be able to offer her much except reassurance that her symptoms probably didn't represent a serious illness. Even as I walked into the room, I would catch myself trying out phrases in advance, variations upon my inevitably disappointing answers to her inevitable questions: "Are you sure this isn't something serious? Isn't there anything you can do?" I was always tempted (and more than once succumbed to the desire) to be definite, to be positive, to be the utterly authoritative healer of my patient's dreams: "Mrs. Smith, you obviously have a bad case of rhinopharyngitis. Take this magic elixir and come see me next Thursday. I'm sure you'll feel better!" Only my fear that somehow she would recognize "rhinopharyngitis" as doctor's lingo for a cold and my suspicion that she might not be better in a week kept me from making this a regular habit.

I am sure that if the time were all accumulated and tallied, I have literally spent days trying to explain the uncertainty of medicine to often understandably unwilling patients. Unless the patient already had significant faith in my competence, I usually left those consultations feeling that she was convinced only of my uncertainty and that she must be wishing she had gone to someone who would have given her more help. Occasionally I have described this process to my wife, expressing my frustration at the feelings of incompetence and mistrust that it so often brought out; and she has sometimes gently (and sometimes not so gently) suggested that perhaps it is my own fault, that people obviously want more assurance and more certainty from their doctor than I am willing to offer, that perhaps I should swallow my "less than five percent probability" and give these patients the reassurance they need to get well.

Laurel Tilson, a close friend, was seeing an obstetrician in Minneapolis prior to the delivery of her first child, and during the last weeks of her pregnancy she developed moderately severe "pregnancy-induced hypertension," or toxemia, a dangerous complication of pregnancy threatening both mother and baby. She described to us how concerned and anxious she was until she asked her doctor if the toxemia could possibly hurt her baby. "Not with me as your doctor," he replied and went on to the next question. "I was so relieved," Laurel said to us later. "I could relax for the rest of the pregnancy knowing that nothing was going to happen to the baby." Everything did turn out all right with her baby, and her obstetrician's self-confidence probably was therapeutic in allowing Laurel to relax and get her needed rest during the last weeks of pregnancy, but the obstetrician certainly was being less than honest about the dangers and uncertainties involved.

Perhaps my wife is right that my patients deserve that kind of reassurance to help them muster their own personal resources in the struggle to get well. For me, however, there is something fundamentally dishonest in such a distortion of the truth. Life is uncertain. The physician who conceals that uncertainty with false reassurances ultimately is robbing the patient of her responsibility for her own life. Although my frustration sometimes leads me to compromise, the moral and emotional consequences of such misrepresentation[9] seem to me too far-reaching to make it a regular part in my practice of medicine.

Chapter 6

MISTAKES

ON A WARM JULY MORNING I finish my rounds at the hospital around nine o'clock and walk across the parking lot to the clinic. After greeting Jackie, I look through the list of my day's appointments and notice that Barb Daily will be in for her first prenatal examination. "Wonderful," I think, recalling the joy of helping her deliver her first child two years ago. Barb and her husband, Russ, had been friends of mine before Heather was born, but we grew much closer with the shared experience of her birth. In a rural family practice such as mine, much of every workday is taken up with disease; I look forward to the prenatal visit with Barb, to the continuing relationship with her over the next months, to the prospect of birth.

At her appointment that afternoon, Barb seems to be in good health, with all the signs and symptoms of pregnancy: slight nausea, some soreness in her breasts, a little weight gain. But when the nurse tests Barb's urine to determine if she is pregnant, the result is negative. The test measures the level of a hormone that is produced by a woman and shows up in her urine when she is pregnant. But occasionally it fails to detect the low levels of the hormone during early pregnancy. I reassure Barb that she is fine and schedule another test for the following week.

Barb leaves a urine sample at the clinic a week later, but the test is negative again. I am troubled. Perhaps she isn't pregnant. Her missed menstrual period and her other symptoms could be a result of a minor hormonal imbalance. Maybe the embryo has died within the uterus and a miscarriage is soon to take place. I could find out by ordering an ultrasound examination. This procedure would give me a "picture" of the uterus and of the embryo. But Barb would have to go to Duluth for the examination. The procedure is also expensive. I know the Dailys well enough to know they have a modest income. Besides, by waiting a few weeks, I should be able to find out for sure without the ultrasound: either the urine test will be positive or Barb will have a miscarriage. I call her and tell her about the negative test result, about the possibility of a miscarriage, and about the necessity of seeing me again if she misses her next menstrual period.

It is, as usual, a hectic summer; I think no more about Barb's troubling state until a month later, when she returns to my office. Nothing has changed: still no menstrual period, still no miscarriage. She is confused and upset. "I feel so pregnant," she tells me. I am bothered, too. Her uterus, upon examination, is slightly enlarged, as it was on the previous visit. But it hasn't grown any larger. Her urine test remains negative. I can think of several possible explanations for her condition, including a hormonal imbalance or even a tumor. But the most likely explanation is that she is carrying a dead embryo. I decide it is time to break the bad news to her.

"I think you have what doctors call a 'missed abortion,'" I tell her. "You were probably pregnant, but the baby appears to have died some weeks ago, before your first examination. Unfortunately, you didn't have a miscarriage to get rid of the dead tissue from the baby and the placenta. If a miscarriage doesn't occur within a few weeks, I'd recommend a re-examination, another pregnancy test, and if nothing shows up, a dilation and curettage procedure to clean out the uterus."

Barb is disappointed; there are tears. She is college-educated, and she understands the scientific and technical aspects of her situation, but that doesn't alleviate the sorrow. We talk at some length and make an appointment for two weeks later.

When Barb returns, Russ is with her. Still no menstrual period; still no miscarriage; still another negative pregnancy test, the fourth. I explain to them what has happened. The dead embryo should be removed or there could be serious complications. Infection could develop; Barb could even become sterile. The conversation is emotionally difficult for all three of us. We schedule the dilation and curettage for later in the week.

Friday morning, Barb is wheeled into the small operating room of the hospital. Barb, the nurses, and I all know one another—it's a small town. The atmosphere is warm and relaxed; we chat before the operation. After Barb is anesthetized, I examine her pelvis again. Her muscles are now completely relaxed, and it is possible to perform a more reliable examination. Her uterus feels bigger than it did two days ago; it is perhaps the size of a small grapefruit. But since all the pregnancy tests were negative and I'm so sure of the diagnosis, I ignore the information from my fingertips and begin the operation.

Dilation and curettage, or D & C, is a relatively simple surgical procedure performed thousands of times each day in this country. First, the cervix is stretched by pushing smooth metal rods of increasing diameter in and out of it. After about five minutes of this, the cervix has expanded enough so that a curette can be inserted through it into the uterus. The curette is another metal rod, at the end of which is an oval ring about an inch at its widest diameter. It is used to scrape the walls of the uterus. The operation is done completely by feel after the cervix has been stretched, since it is still too narrow to see through.

Things do not go easily this morning. There is considerably more blood than usual, and it is only with great difficulty that I am able to extract anything. What should take ten or fifteen minutes stretches into a half-hour. The body parts I remove are much larger than I expected, considering when the embryo died. They are not bits of decomposing tissue. These are parts of a body that was recently alive!

I do my best to suppress my rising panic and try to complete the procedure. Working blindly, I am unable to evacuate the uterus completely; I can feel more parts inside but cannot remove them. Finally I stop, telling myself that the uterus will expel the rest within a few days.

Russ is waiting outside the operating room. I tell him that Barb is fine but that there were some problems with the operation. Since I don't completely understand what happened, I can't be very helpful in answering his questions. I promise to return to the hospital later in the day after Barb has awakened from the anesthesia.

In between seeing other patients that morning, I place several almost frantic phone calls, trying to piece together what happened. Despite reassurances from a pathologist that it is "impossible" for a pregnant woman to have four consecutive negative pregnancy tests, the realization is growing that I have aborted Barb's living child. I won't know for sure until the pathologist has examined the fetal parts and determined the baby's age and the cause of death. In a daze, I walk over to the hospital and tell Russ and Barb as much as I know for sure without letting them know all I suspect. I tell them that more tissue may be expelled. I can't face my own suspicions.

Two days later, on Sunday morning, I receive a tearful call from Barb. She has just passed some recognizable body parts; what is she to do? She tells me that the bleeding has stopped now and that she feels better. The abortion I began on Friday is apparently over. I set up an appointment to meet with her and Russ to review the entire situation.

The pathologist's report confirms my worst fears: I aborted a living fetus. It was about eleven weeks old. I can find no one who can explain why Barb had four negative pregnancy tests. My meeting with Barb and Russ later in the week is one of the hardest things I have ever been through. I described in some detail what I did and what my rationale had been. Nothing can obscure the hard reality: I killed their baby.

Politely, almost meekly, Russ asks whether the ultrasound examination would have shown that Barb was carrying a live baby. It almost seems that he is trying to protect my feelings, trying to absolve me of some of the responsibility. "Yes," I answer, "if I had ordered the ultrasound, we would have known the baby was alive." I cannot explain why I didn't recommend it.

Mistakes are an inevitable part of everyone's life. They happen; they hurt—ourselves and others. They demonstrate our fallibility. Shown our mistakes and forgiven them, we can grow, perhaps in some small way become better people. Mistakes, understood this way, are a process, a way we connect with one another and with our deepest selves.

But mistakes seem different for doctors. This has to do with the very nature of our work. A mistake in the intensive care unit, in the emergency room, in the surgery suite, or at the sickbed is different from a mistake on the dock or at the typewriter. A doctor's miscalculation or oversight can prolong an illness, or cause a permanent disability, or kill a patient. Few other mistakes are more costly.

Developments in modern medicine have provided doctors with more knowledge of the human body, more accurate methods of diagnosis, more sophisticated technology to help in examining and monitoring the sick. All of that means more power to intervene in the disease process. But modern medicine, with its invasive tests and potentially lethal drugs, has also given doctors the power to do more harm.

Yet precisely because of its technological wonders and near-miraculous drugs, modern medicine has created for the physician an expectation of perfection. The technology seems so exact that error becomes almost unthinkable. We are not prepared for our mistakes, and we don't know how to cope with them when they occur. Doctors are not alone in harboring expectations of perfection. Patients, too, expect doctors to be perfect. Perhaps patients have to consider their doctors less prone to error than other people: how else can a sick or injured person, already afraid, come to trust the doctor? Further, modern medicine has taken much of the treatment of illness out of the realm of common sense; a patient must trust a physician to make decisions that he, the patient, only vaguely understands. But the degree of perfection expected by patients is no doubt also a result of what we doctors have come to believe about ourselves, or better, have tried to convince ourselves about ourselves.

This perfection is a grand illusion, of course, a game of mirrors that everyone plays. Doctors hide their mistakes from patients, from other doctors, even from themselves. Open discussion of mistakes is banished from the consultation room, from the operating room, from physicians' meetings. Mistakes become gossip, and are spoken of openly only in court. Unable to admit our mistakes, we physicians are cut off from healing. We cannot ask for forgiveness, and we get none. We are thwarted, stunted; we do not grow.

During the days, and weeks, and months after I aborted Barb's baby, my guilt and anger grew. I did discuss what had happened with my partners, with the pathologist, with obstetric specialists. Some of my mistakes were obvious: I had relied too heavily on one test; I had not been skillful in determining the size of the uterus by pelvic examination; I should have ordered the ultrasound before proceeding to the D & C. There was no way I could justify what I had done. To make matters worse, there were complications following the D & C, and Barb was unable to become pregnant again for two years.

Although I was as honest with the Dailys as I could have been, and although I told them everything they wanted to know, I never shared with them my own agony. I felt they had enough sorrow without having to bear my burden as well. I decided it was my responsibility to deal with my guilt alone. I never asked for their forgiveness. Doctors' mistakes, of course, come in a variety of packages and stem from a variety of causes. For primary care practitioners, who see every kind of problem from cold sores to cancer, the mistakes are often simply a result of not knowing enough. One evening during my years in Minnesota a local boy was brought into the emergency room after a drunken driver had knocked him off his bicycle. I examined him right away. Aside from swelling and bruising of the left leg and foot, he seemed fine. An x-ray showed what appeared to be a dislocation of the foot from the ankle. I consulted by telephone with an orthopedic specialist in Duluth, and we decided that I could operate on the boy. As was my usual practice, I offered the patient and his mother (who happened to be a nurse with whom I worked regularly) a choice: I could do the operation or they could travel to Duluth to see the specialist. My pride was hurt when she decided to take her son to Duluth.

My feelings changed considerably when the specialist called the next morning to thank me for the referral. He reported that the boy had actually suffered an unusual muscle injury, a posterior compartment syndrome, which had twisted his foot and caused it to appear to be dislocated. I had never even heard of such a syndrome, much less seen or treated it. The boy had required immediate surgery to save the muscles of his lower leg. Had his mother not decided to take him to Duluth, he would have been permanently disabled.

Sometimes a lack of technical skill leads to a mistake. After I had been in town a few years, the doctor who had done most of the surgery at the clinic left to teach at a medical school. Since the clinic was more than a hundred miles from the nearest surgical center, my partners and I decided that I should get some additional training in order to be able to perform emergency surgery. One of my first cases after training was a young man with appendicitis. The surgery proceeded smoothly enough, but the patient did not recover as quickly as he should have, and his hemoglobin level (a measure of the amount of blood in the system) dropped slowly. I referred him to a surgeon in Duluth, who, during a second operation, found a significant amount of old blood in his abdomen. Apparently I had left a small blood vessel leaking into the abdominal cavity. Perhaps I hadn't noticed the oozing blood during surgery; perhaps it had begun to leak only after I had finished. Although the young man was never in serious danger, although the blood vessel would probably have sealed itself without the second surgery, my mistake had caused considerable discomfort and added expense.

Often, I am sure, mistakes are a result of simple carelessness. There was the young girl I treated for what I thought was a minor ankle injury. After looking at her x-rays, I sent her home with what I diagnosed as a sprain. A radiologist did a routine follow-up review of the x-rays and sent me a report. I failed to read it carefully and did not notice that her ankle had been broken. I first learned about my mistake five years later when I was summoned to a court hearing. The fracture I had missed had not healed properly, and the patient had required extensive treatment and difficult surgery. By that time I couldn't even remember her original visit and had to piece together what had happened from my records.

Some mistakes are purely technical; most involve a failure of judgment. Perhaps the worst kind involve what another physician has described to me as "a failure of will." She was referring to those situations in which a doctor knows the right thing to do but doesn't do it because he is distracted, or pressured, or exhausted.

Several years ago, I was rushing down the hall of the hospital to the delivery room. A young woman stopped me. Her mother had been having chest pains all night. Should she be brought to the emergency room? I knew the mother well, had examined her the previous week, and knew of her recurring bouts of chest pains. She suffered from angina; I presumed she was having another attack.

Some part of me knew that anyone with all-night chest pains should be seen right away. But I was under pressure. The delivery would make me an hour late to the office, and I was frayed from a weekend on call, spent mostly in the emergency room. This new demand would mean additional pressure. "No," I said, "take her over to the office, and I'll see her as soon as I'm done here." About twenty minutes later, as I was finishing the delivery, the clinic nurse rushed into the room. Her face was pale. "Come quick! Mrs. Helgeson just collapsed." I sprinted the hundred yards to the office, where I found Mrs. Helgeson in cardiac arrest. Like many doctors' offices at the time, ours did not have the advanced life-support equipment that helps keep patients alive long enough to get them to a hospital. Despite everything we did, Mrs. Helgeson died.

Would she have survived if I had agreed to see her in the emergency room, where the requisite staff and equipment were available? No one will ever know for sure. But I have to live with the possibility that she might not have died if I had not had "a failure of will." There was no way to rationalize it: I had been irresponsible, and a patient had died.

Many situations do not lend themselves to a simple determination of whether a mistake has been made. Seriously ill, hospitalized patients, for instance, require of doctors almost continuous decision-making. Although in most cases no single mistakes is obvious, there always seem to be things that could have been done differently or better: administering more of this medication, starting that treatment a little sooner....The fact is that when a patient dies, the physician is left wondering whether the care he provided was adequate. There is no way to be certain, for it is impossible to determine what would have happened if things had been done differently. Often it is difficult to get an honest opinion on this even from another physician, most doctors not wanting to be perceived by their colleagues as judgmental—or perhaps fearing similar judgments upon themselves. In the end, the physician has to suppress the guilt and move on to the next patient.

A few years after my mistake with Barb Daily, Maiya Martinen first came to see me halfway through her pregnancy. I did not know her or her husband well, but I knew that they were solid, hard-working people. This was to be their first child. When I examined Maiya, it seemed to me that the fetus was unusually small, and I was uncertain about her due date. I sent her to Duluth for an ultrasound examination—which was by now routine for almost any problem during pregnancy—and an evaluation by an obstetrician. The obstetrician thought the baby would be small, but he thought it could be safely delivered in the local hospital.

Maiya's labor was uneventful, except that it took her longer than usual to push the baby through to delivery. Her baby boy was born blue and floppy, but he responded well to routine newborn resuscitation measures. Fifteen minutes after birth, however, he had a short seizure. We checked his blood sugar level and found it to be low, a common cause of seizures in small babies who take longer than usual to emerge from the birth canal. Fortunately, we were able to put an IV easily into a scalp vein and administer glucose, and baby Marko seemed to improve. He and his mother were discharged from the hospital several days later.

At about two months of age, a few days after I had given him his first set of immunizations, Marko began having short spells. Not long after that he started to have full-blown seizures. Once again the Martinens made the trip to Duluth, and Marko was hospitalized for three days of tests. No cause for the seizures was found, but he was placed on medication. Marko continued to have seizures, however. When he returned for his second set of immunizations, it was clear to me that he was not doing well.

The remainder of Marko's short life was a tribute to the faith and courage of his parents. He proved severely retarded, and the seizures became harder and harder to control. Maiya eventually went East for a few months so Marko could be treated at the National Institutes of Health. But nothing seemed to help, and Maiya and her baby returned home. Marko had to be admitted frequently to the local hospital in order to control his seizures. At two o'clock one morning I was called to the hospital: the baby had had a respiratory arrest. Despite our efforts, Marko died, ending a year-and-a-half struggle with life.

No cause for Marko's condition was ever determined. Did something happen during the birth that briefly cut off oxygen to his brain? Should Maiya have delivered at the high-risk obstetric center in Duluth, where sophisticated fetal monitoring is available? Should I have sent Marko to the Newborn Intensive Care Unit in Duluth immediately after his first seizure in the delivery room? I subsequently learned that children who have seizures should not routinely be immunized. Would it have made any difference if I had never given Marko the shots? There were many such questions in my mind and, I am sure, in the minds of the Martinens. There was no way to know the answers, no way for me to handle the guilt feelings I experienced, perhaps irrationally, whenever I saw Maiya.

The emotional consequences of mistakes are difficult enough to handle. But soon after I started practicing I realized I had to face another anxiety as well: it is not only in the emergency room, the operating room, the intensive care unit, or the delivery room that a doctor can blunder into tragedy. Errors are always possible, even in the midst of the humdrum routine of daily care. Was that baby with diarrhea more dehydrated than he looked, and should I have hospitalized him? Will that nine-year-old with stomach cramps whose mother I just lectured about psychosomatic illness end up in the operating room tomorrow with a ruptured appendix? Did that Vietnamese refugee have a problem I didn't understand because of the language barrier? A doctor has to confront the possibility of a mistake with every patient visit.

My initial response to the mistakes I did make was to question my competence. Perhaps I just didn't have the necessary intelligence, judgment, and discipline to be a physician. But was I really incompetent? My University of Minnesota Medical School class had voted me one of the two most promising clinicians. My diploma from the National Board of Medical Examiners showed scores well above average. I knew that the townspeople considered me a good physician; I knew that my partners, with whom I worked daily, and the consultants to whom I referred patients considered me a good physician, too. When I looked at it objectively, my competence was not the issue. I would have to learn to live with my mistakes.

A physician is even less prepared to deal with his mistakes than is the average person. Nothing in our training prepares us to respond appropriately. As a student, I was simply not aware that the sort of mistakes I would eventually make in practice actually happened to competent physicians. As far as I can remember from my student experience on the hospital wards, the only doctors who ever made mistakes were the much maligned "LMDs"— local medical doctors. They would transfer their patients who weren't doing well to the University Hospital. At the "U," teams of specialist physicians with their residents, interns, and students would take their turns examining the patient thoroughly, each one delighted to discover (in retrospect, of course) an "obvious" error made by the referring LMD. As students we had the entire day to evaluate and care for our five to ten patients. After we examined them and wrote orders for their care, first the interns and then the residents would also examine them and correct our orders. Finally, the supervising physician would review everything. It was pretty unlikely that a major error would slip by; and if it did, it could always be blamed on someone else on the team. We had very little feeling for what it was like to be the LMD, working alone with perhaps the same number of hospital patients plus an office full of other patients; but we were quite sure we would not be guilty of such grievous errors as we saw coming into the U.

An atmosphere of precision pervaded the teaching hospital. The uncertainty that came to seem inescapable to me in northern Minnesota would shrivel away at the U as teams of specialists pronounced authoritatively upon any subject. And when a hospital physician did make a significant mistake, it was first whispered about the halls as if it were a sin. Much later a conference would be called in which experts who had had weeks to think about the case would discuss the way it should have been handled. The embarrassing mistake was frequently not even mentioned; it had evaporated. One could almost believe that the patient had been treated perfectly. More important, only the technical aspects of the case were considered relevant for discussion. It all seemed so simple, so clear. How could anyone do anything else? There was no mention of the mistake, or of the feelings of the patient or the doctor. It was hardly the sort of environment in which a doctor might feel free to talk about his mistakes or about his emotional responses to them.

Medical school was also a very competitive place, discouraging any sharing of feelings. The favorite pastime, even between classes or at a party, seemed to be sharing with the other medical students the story of the patient who had been presented to one's team, and then describing in detail how the diagnosis had been reached, how the disease worked, and what the treatment was. The story-teller, having spent the day researching every detail of the patient's disease, could, of course, dazzle everyone with the breadth and depth of his knowledge. Even though I knew what was going on, the game still left me feeling incompetent, as it must have many of my colleagues. I never knew for sure, though, since no one had the nerve to say so. It almost seemed that one's peers were the worst possible persons with whom to share those feelings.

Physicians in private practice are no more likely to find errors openly acknowledged or discussed, even though they occur regularly. My own mistakes represent only some of those of which I am aware. I know of one physician who administered a potent drug in a dose ten times that recommended; his patient almost died. Another doctor examined a child in an emergency room late one night and told the parents the problem was only a mild viral infection. Only because the parents did not believe the doctor, only because they consulted another doctor the following morning, did the child survive a life-threatening infection. Still another physician killed a patient while administering a routine test: a needle slipped and lacerated a vital artery. Whether the physician is a rural general practitioner with years of experience but only basic training or a recently graduated, highly trained neurosurgeon working in a sophisticated technological environment, the basic problem is the same.

Because doctors do not discuss their mistakes, I do not know how other physicians come to terms with theirs. But I suspect that many cannot bear to face their mistakes directly. We either deny the misfortune altogether or blame the patient, the nurse, the laboratory, other physicians, the system, fate—anything to avoid our own guilt.

The medical profession seems to have no place for its mistakes. Indeed, one would almost think that mistakes were sins. And if the medical profession has no room for doctors' mistakes, neither does society. The number of malpractice suits filed each year is symptomatic of this. In what other profession are practitioners regularly sued for hundreds of thousands of dollars because of misjudgments? I am sure the Dailys could have successfully sued me for a large amount of money had they chosen to do so.

The drastic consequences of our mistakes, the repeated opportunities to make them, the uncertainty about our culpability, and the professional denial that mistakes happen all work together to create an intolerable dilemma for the physician. We see the horror or our mistakes, yet we cannot deal with their enormous emotional impact.

Perhaps the only way to face our guilt is through confession, restitution, and absolution. Yet within the structure of modern medicine there is no place for such spiritual healing. Although the emotionally mature physician may be able to give the patient or family a full description of what happened, the technical details are often so difficult for the layperson to understand that the nature of the mistake is hidden. If an error is clearly described, it is frequently presented as "natural," "understandable," or "unavoidable" (which, indeed, it often is). But there is seldom a real confession: "This is the mistake I made; I'm sorry." How can one say that to a grieving parent? to a woman who has lost her mother?

If confession is difficult, what are we to say about restitution? The very nature of a physician's work means that there are things that cannot be restored in any meaningful way. What could I do to make good the Dailys' loss?

I have not been successful in dealing with a paradox: I am a healer, yet I sometimes do more harm than good. Obviously, we physicians must do everything we can to keep mistakes to a minimum. But if we are unable to deal openly with those that do occur, we will find neurotic ways to protect ourselves from the pain we feel. Little wonder that physicians are accused of playing God. Little wonder that we are defensive about our judgments, that we blame the patient or the previous physician when things go wrong, that we yell at nurses for their mistakes, that we have such high rates of alcoholism, drug addiction, and suicide.

At some point we must all bring medical mistakes out of the closet. This will be difficult as long as both the profession and society continue to project their desires for perfection onto the doctor. Physicians need permission to admit errors. They need permission to share them with their patients. The practice of medicine is difficult enough without having to bear the yoke of perfection.

Chapter 7

TAKING SIDES

IT IS A LATE summer Saturday night, almost Sunday morning, when the phone rings. Tourist season, so I'm not surprised.

"Dr. Hilfiker? This is Grace down at the emergency room. We have a patient for you again."

"OK, what's the problem?" I suppose it doesn't really matter, but I like to prepare myself on the way down the hill for whatever awaits me. Since it's Saturday night, I can almost guess.

"It's John Maynor. He's been in an accident. Got a pretty deep gash on his forehead, but he seems OK otherwise. I guess he's been drinking."

I sigh. "All right. I'm on my way. Are the police there yet?"

"They brought him in, and they're talking to him now."

"OK. See you in a minute."

I try for the thousandth time to estimate the cost of alcohol to our society. It seems to me that 90 percent of the Friday and Saturday night calls involve alcohol in some way—accidents, of course, but also spouse abuse and psychiatric emergencies. Even the patients coming to the emergency room with the usual range of physical complaints might not be there at all if it weren't for alcohol: the child with the minor illness whose intoxicated parents' judgment has been impaired; the drunk with a cold who decides he has to get it checked out right now; the chronic alcoholic with serious pneumonia.

My thoughts return to John Maynor. Ordinarily, I quite enjoy the suturing of minor wounds, but I don't look forward to dealing with John when he's drunk. He and I have been through this before. I think he actually likes me when he's sober, but he won't like anybody tonight. I try to steel myself for the ordeal.

Bob Nixon, one-third of our total police force, is waiting for me outside the doors of the emergency room. "Hi, Doc. I guess Grace told you we brought Johnny in again. He fell asleep coming into town and went into the ditch. Out cold when we found him. We're going to throw the book at him this time. Can you get us a blood sample?"

"Yeah, sure. Wait till I'm done fixing him up." The police need a blood sample to document his intoxication, but I don't like being the one to provide it. It sets me against John right from the start and ruins whatever rapport might develop. So I shove it to last on the agenda.

"Doc, you get me outta here!" John howls at me even before I'm through the emergency-room door. "It's just a scratch, and I don't need no goddamn doctor. You tell that fuckin' Nixon I don't need to be here. I ain't payin' for this, ya know. That fuckin' cop brought me in here." John is sitting up on the exam table, blood streaming from the left side of his forehead. Grace Maki is running back and forth in front of him, trying to hold a compress on the wound as John bobs from side to side. Forty-five years old, ruggedly handsome, a chronic alcoholic, John is a small-town tragedy. The only times I see him sober are when he has to spend a few days in the hospital or jail or when we force him into our outpatient alcoholism treatment program for a few weeks.

"Let me look at your head, John. That cut looks pretty nasty." I wait for him to give me some sign I can proceed. Usually if I can avoid forcing the issue, even someone as belligerently drunk as John will settle down and let me work. Besides, I'm concerned he might have a concussion, and I don't want him walking out before I can evaluate him.

"Oh no ya don't, Doc. Last time this cost me two hunnert bucks, and I ain't payin' this time. Let me go home." He starts to get off the cart. I'm always amazed at John's tolerance for alcohol. Last time we measured his blood alcohol at 0.32 percent, enough to render most people unconscious, but John's speech was barely slurred. He just gets unpleasant.

"John, I'm not going to force you to do anything. But that cut looks pretty bad to me. I'm worried you might have hurt your head in the accident. I'd suggest you let me take a look."

"What accident...?" He looks at me, the belligerence melting into confused fear. "I wasn't in no accident! Those fuckin' cops came and got me....What accident?"

I was afraid of this. Although he might only be suffering an alcoholic blackout, John probably has temporary amnesia from a concussion.

"Bob says you ran your car off the road. Don't you remember?"

"Hell no! I was down at my brother's when those cops...I don't know, but I wasn't in no accident."

"Well, let me take a look at your forehead there." John is frightened enough now to be more accommodating. He lies down and promptly falls asleep. Though bleeding profusely, his laceration is not difficult to repair. Rousing him twenty minutes later, I ask enough questions to determine that he probably has had a concussion and should stay in the hospital for observation. I examine him briefly to rule out serious brain damage, but in his condition a full examination is out of the question.

Next we come to the blood alcohol. "John, Bob wants me to draw a blood test—"

"No fuckin' way."

"Well, that's between you and Bob. I told you I wasn't going to force you into anything. I'll call Bob back in." I let the police officer from the waiting area and leave while he covers the legal formalities with John. I have a hunch I might have to see John quite a bit as a patient, and I don't want to destroy whatever relationship we have by appearing to side with the police.

Ten minutes later, after arranging for John's admission to the hospital, I return to find Bob intoning to a now sleeping John the required statement concerning the legal implications of his having refused the blood test. I step outside the room until Bob is finished and then try to wake my patient up again.

"John, I think you'd better stay in the hospital for a day or two. Apparently you were knocked out during the accident, and I'm afraid you might have some brain damage."

"What accident? I wasn't in no fuckin' accident. An' I ain't stayin' in no hospital. Who the hell d'ya think is gonna pay for a hospital?"

It isn't easy, but I finally convince John that he has to stay for observation. "I think we should get some tests, too," I say. "Just to be sure."

"What kinda tests?"

"Oh, some x-rays of your head, and a blood test."

"What kinda blood test?"

I want to test the level of alcohol in John's blood to make sure his confusion and stupor are from intoxication and not head injury. My mind flits back to a Sunday morning some years ago when I hospitalized an "obvious" drunk after an accident, only to discover some hours later that his blood alcohol level was almost zero and his stupor was the result of head injury. I don't think I can explain to John the difference between a blood test drawn for legal reasons and one drawn for medical reasons, so I parry his question: "Just some tests to make sure nothing else is wrong, John."

"Wait a minute. Is this something Nixon thought up to get that blood from me? What are you guys up to?"

"Nothing, John. I just want to check you over so you'll be all right." Actually, the "medical blood alcohol" and the "legal blood alcohol" are the same tests, but the latter is handled by the state highway patrol laboratory to make sure the results will be valid in court. Since our hospital records can always be subpoenaed, however, the distinction between the tests is a bit fuzzy at best. In fact, everything that becomes a part of John's medical record could be subpoenaed, so he has every reason to be suspicious. Only by vigorously threatening him with the potential health consequences of his refusal, and promising him that "Nixon will never see the tests," do I cajole John into accepting our evaluation and hospitalization.

The next morning John is awake and shaven when I come in for hospital rounds. His concussion turns out to have been minor (I can't even be sure that all his symptoms weren't the direct result of alcohol), and he is anxious to go home. However, his sister, Christine Marshall, and our local alcoholism counselor, Mary Rudd, have been discussing the possibility of commitment to a long-term treatment unit where John would be confined for at least six months in an attempt to deal with his alcoholism. John has no close family, no regular job that he needs to be sober for, and no nondrinking friends—none of the factors that might encourage him to take a treatment program seriously—so I'm not very optimistic about the ability of such a program to change him. But as I can think of no other alternative to his gradual slide into an early death, I agree to do what I can. I return to his room.

"Christine and Mary think you ought to go down to Moose Lake for a while, John, to see if you can't get this drinking under control. I think you ought to give it a try."

"Doc, that ain't gonna do no good. You know me better than that." He looks up at me and grins. John is that curious mixture of integrity and con, honesty and swindle, so disarming in many alcoholics. "You know I'm gonna drink myself to death. The Cure ain't gonna do nothin' for me. Just let me go my own way, huh?"

"If I let you go this morning, you'll just get drunk again, right?"

"Prob'ly, Doc. That's what usually happens, ain't it?"

"Well, I told Christine I'd keep you here a couple of days until things clear up and we can talk more about this. I hope you'll stay voluntarily, John, but if you won't I'll sign a seventy-two-hour hold on you!"

Beneath the con, I can see the anger rising in John's eyes. He knows he's trapped, and he's too street-wise to fight when he's outnumbered. I never actually have to sign the hold order, but John's hospital stay is anything but voluntary, and the commitment proceedings are messy. John hires an out-of-town lawyer and tries to fight. Eventually I have to testify at his hearing about my many contacts with John, about the evidence for alcoholism in his examination and lab tests, and about my belief that he is indeed an alcoholic. I try to convince myself that I am still acting in John's best interest, but the lines are, to say the least, fuzzy. I'm certainly not testifying "on his behalf." I wonder what our next contacts will be like, whether he'll follow my advice to stay at the hospital, whether he'll trust me with anything. Whose side am I on, anyway?

John's situation placed me in conflict with a key medical principle: physicians are to work as agents of their patients. Although this ethical principle may not be stated explicitly, it is assumed by patients and physicians alike. Patients see their physicians as their healers and confidants, and entrust them with information they would reveal to no one else. Physician training in medical school and postgraduate education emphasizes the primacy of the patient. The physician's personal advantage, the good of society, the interests of others, are all to be subordinated to the interests of the patient. The physician is to ally herself with the patient, in a sense to identify with the patient, to see the world through his eyes and seek only his advantage. Even the economic structure of the medical encounter emphasizes this principle: The physician is theoretically hired by the patient and becomes, for that moment in time, his employee.

Because of my own inclinations, training, and experience, I found it very important to see myself as my patients' agent. In many cases I entered so deeply into their lives that I saw myself almost as their extension, fighting perhaps against family, employer, or bureaucracy to secure what was important for their health. How broadly I was to extend this principle was never defined. Thus, when I violated it by, say, drawing a legal blood alcohol for the purpose of convicting my patient of drunken driving, I felt guilty of betrayal.

In John's case and others like it, I could usually convince myself that I was acting in the patient's ultimate interest and was not really compromising my personal commitment to him. There were other occasions, however, in which I was more clearly acting as society's agent against my patient. When Roger Tuttle came into the office with a form from the Social Security Administration, he wanted me to help him get Social Security benefits because of his back injury. Roger had been a self-employed logger until a tree he was felling pinned him to the ground.

Although no bones were broken, his back was never the same. He tried several times to return to work, but the heavy lifting required by his job kept reinjuring his back. He suffered for several years with chronic back pain and was unable to find work.

When I filled out a disability form, however, I was acting not as Roger's advocate but as an impartial agent for the Social Security Administration to determine whether he was sufficiently disabled to merit compensation. Although disability examinations are occasionally clear-cut (if you've lost a leg, you've lost a leg), most are like Roger's. They deal with imprecise quantities—emotional disability, weakness due to heart failure, back pain. For the purpose of calculating the amount of compensation, a single number—the disability percentage—is computed. In these examinations I was no longer simply working to help my patient. Rather, I became judge and jury, trying to elicit information that would allow me to form an impartial judgment about the disability.

Like Roger, most patients applying to me for disability were also my patients. Often they correctly perceived the adversarial nature of our relationship and initially tried to behave accordingly; but I performed the interview and examination in the same way I usually did, asking all the same questions. Because of the trust we had previously developed, the patient would normally end up answering frankly, just as if this were an ordinary examination. But it wasn't. In fact, the interview and examination were a sort of informal court proceeding—but without the patient having the advantage of a lawyer or even of a clearly stated adversarial relationship. In the guise of friend, advocate, and personal physician, I was gathering information that would be used to make a judgment for society against my patient. (I am not implying that patients usually wanted to lie or distort the truth about their condition; rather, the questions raised on the form were often subtle ones on which there could be legitimate differences of opinion—alcohol use, emotional stability, or the extent to which an illness actually interfered in the patient's functioning.) Even if the patient did succeed in stonewalling the proceedings, I still had access (either in my records or in my memory) to other visits during which he had assumed I was there only to help him. All of the disability forms required me, as a physician, to disclose whether I had any other information bearing on the question.

The disability examination, however, was only a particularly glaring example of society's demand that I compromise my role as patient advocate. The insurance physical, the pre-employment examination, even the examination after a prolonged illness to determine fitness to return to work, all were instances in which I became society's representative making a judgment for the good of some segment of that society—the insurance company, the employer, and so on. The subtle but very definite change in perspective which accompanied these encounters did damage to the physician-patient relationship by engendering mutual feelings of suspicion and creating in me worries that my patients might be manipulating me, or I them.

The question of where my loyalties lay became even more distressing to me when I discovered during the course of caring for a patient that his condition should limit some socially permitted privilege. Walter Moffatt, for instance, was a delightful elderly man who had been a devoted patient of mine for a number of years. (My practice style and personality did not encourage "devoted" patients, but Walter had been impressed years ago by a thorough physical I gave him, and had been a real source of joy for me ever since.) He was a vigorous, staunchly independent man who prided himself on his driving ability as he neared ninety years old. As I saw him regularly, however, it became clear that his intellectual faculties were slipping badly and he was becoming forgetful. Through the grapevine I heard several reports of near accidents, situations in which Walter's judgment had not been up to par. Finally, one of our public health nurses asked if I couldn't do something.

At Walter's next physical, I came to the conclusion that he should not be driving. Not only was his judgment deteriorating, but his hearing and vision were failing too. As supportively as possible, I told him I thought he should no longer drive. He was obviously offended, but he promised to follow my advice since he "trusted me so much." Several weeks later, however, he was still driving, so I decided to notify the state licensing bureau of my concern. Walter's license was withdrawn. It could be argued that I had done what was best for Walter, but one is easily led by such arguments into arrogance and condescension toward one's patients. In Walter's case, although I had told him in advance of my intentions, he was angered and hurt by my action. He did not visit me for another year, by which time his senility had progressed to the point where I believe he had forgotten the incident.

The physician's legal responsibility to report certain crimes is another example of how the physician-patient relationship can be drastically altered by the needs of society. In Minnesota, for example, spouse abuse and child abuse must be reported to the proper authorities by any physician who has reason even to suspect their presence. This is a very sensible law, intended for the benefit, ultimately, of everyone. It did, however, set me against my patients. I could not truthfully reassure them of complete confidentiality, for if they told me "the wrong things" I was obligated to report them.

The authority invested in the physician to order laboratory tests, admit to the hospital, or prescribe medications also provides numerous opportunities for the physician to come into conflict with his patients' goals. Martha Muldoon is one of my few "regulars." Sixty-five years old, wife of a chronically ill man, Martha is thin, almost emaciated, and smokes cigarettes constantly. She has diabetes, high blood pressure, and a chronic anxiety that has threatened her ability to cope. We see each other every three or four weeks, just to help keep Martha from falling apart.

"Dr. Hilfiker, you've got to do something for me, or I'm not going to make it. I've almost passed out a couple of times in the past two weeks. That high blood pressure medicine makes me feel weak, and that diabetic diet just doesn't give me enough food to keep up my strength. You know how it is, trying to take care of Bill by myself. I'm not going to make it. You've got to do something for me."

Inwardly I sigh. It's March, and I know how the long Minnesota winter affects Martha. Last year, at this time, I put her in the hospital against my better judgment just to "do something for her," and she drove the nurses crazy for six weeks before I could get her to leave. Just as one symptom would resolve itself and she would be on the verge of checking out, another would appear, demanding evaluation. Her symptoms today are the same ones she had three weeks ago and three weeks before that. She's been hospitalized so that they can be checked on and then followed closely at home by the public health nurse, but none of us have ever found much that we could help. In desperation, I've even tried antidepressant medication, but her symptoms persist. I encourage Martha to talk. I examine her. I suggest some minor changes in her medical regimen, mostly to satisfy her need to "do something." But it doesn't seem to be enough.

"Dr. Hilfiker, why can't you put me in the hospital like you did last year? You know I can't take care of Bill like this. I felt so much better in the hospital. Medicare will cover it, and we've got good insurance besides."

She's right about not being able to take care of her husband. For several years she and Bill have been able to stay in their small home only because of an intensive support network of friends and various helping professionals: hot lunches from the senior center, twice-weekly visits by the public health nurse, twice-weekly visits by the county homemaking service, groceries delivered by friends, rides to town or to Duluth provided by friends. Martha and Bill's life is a miracle of rural cooperation, but even this framework is a delicate one, supported only by their continuing health. If there were any further deterioration in either one, they would both have to come into the nursing home.

The nursing home! As for many older people in our community, the nursing home remains for Martha a symbol of giving up, of death. She was forced to stay there with Bill for a few months some years ago after she injured her back, but she has stubbornly resisted it ever since. She would welcome a hospital stay, but the nursing home is not an option as far as she is concerned. Even when I assure her it would only be temporary, she will hear none of it. If I won't put her in the hospital, then she'll just go home.

Although Martha would like to be in the hospital, her medical needs do not really justify her admission. It would not be difficult to stretch the truth a bit in order to persuade her insurance carriers to pay the bill; but she does not need to be in the hospital. It is, of course, impossible to impress Martha with the logic of this. She knows she doesn't feel well, knows there is room in the hospital (our small county hospital is rarely full), and knows I'll be able to prevail upon her various insurance carriers to cover the bill. Indeed, the inconsistencies of her insurance policies make it less expensive to her to stay in the hospital than in the much cheaper nursing home.

The vagaries of modern medical economics make me the only obstacle between Martha and a long rest in the hospital. There is really nothing else preventing her admission except my conviction that her hospitalization would be an inappropriate use of medical resources. Even our hospital administrator would be happy to have Martha's admission increase his census, but it is, unfortunately, my responsibility to see that medical resources are used wisely. If all the Marthas of the world were admitted to the hospital whenever they didn't feel well, either the system would collapse or everyone's insurance premiums would skyrocket. I am the only effective keeper of the gate.

It is impossible to explain this to Martha. She immediately begins to cry. "You just don't believe me that I'm sick, Dr. Hilfiker. How am I going to take care of Bill at home? I've almost passed out a couple of times in the past two weeks." She begins for the third time in twenty minutes to tell me her symptoms.

"Mrs. Muldoon," I interrupt her, "I can't admit you to the hospital. Let's try reducing your blood pressure medicine a little bit and see if that helps you."

"I don't think that's going to help, Doctor, but I'll do what you say. You know I trust you. I'll make an appointment for two weeks from now, and we'll see if I'm any better."

Martha and I will go through this again, but for the time being I have stood my ground.

It may be argued that in Martha's situation (and also in insurance examinations, limiting driving privileges, or reporting abuse), I am still acting in the ultimate interest of the patient and therefore should feel no real conflict. This argument, however, ignores the long-term adversarial relationship thereby created between two people, doctor and patient, who may be seeing each other for years to come in various critical situations where trust will be essential. The patient is no longer doing his best to give me as much information as possible about himself; rather, he is seeking to persuade me to his own point of view. No longer am I seeking to offer the patient what he desires but that which is in his best interest, or worse, that which is in society's best interest. There is no longer collaboration between patient and physician to arrive at a mutually agreed-upon goal. Each party is working for his or her own purposes.

Chapter 8

PLAYING GOD

THE PHONE RINGS, PULLING me from that deepest sleep which comes during the first hours of the night. I can barely remember who I am, much less why the phone might be ringing. I manage to find the receiver next to the bed and pick it up.

"Hello?"

"Hello, Dr. Hilfiker? This is Ginger at the nursing home. Elsa has a fever."

In the silence my mind is immediately clear. Elsa Toivonen, eighty-three years old, confined to the nursing home ever since her stroke three years ago, bedridden, mute. In an instant I remember her as she was before the stroke: her dislike and distrust of doctors and hospitals, her staunch pride and independence despite the crippling back curvature of scoliosis, her wry grin every time I suggested hospitalization for some problem. I remember admitting her to the hospital after her stroke, incontinent, reduced to helplessness, one side completely paralyzed, speech gone; and I remember those first few days during which I aggressively treated the pneumonia that developed as a complication of the stroke, giving her intravenous antibiotics despite her apparent desire to die. "Depressed," I had thought. "She'll get over it. Besides, she may recover substantially in the next few weeks." She did, in fact, recover from the pneumonia, but she remained paralyzed and without speech. For the last three years she has lain curled in her nursing-home bed, my own grim reminder of the power of modern medicine.

"Dr. Hilfiker?" Ginger Moss's voice brings me back to my tired body.

"Oh...yeah," I say. My mind is focused; I just can't get my mouth to work. "Any other symptoms?"

"Well, you know Elsa. It's hard to tell. She hasn't been eating much the last few days, and she's had a little cough. Mary noticed her temp on the evening shift, but she didn't want to bother you."

"So why are you bothering me now?" I want to say. Instead I ask, "What's her temperature?"

"One hundred three point five, rectally."

"Oh…all right," I say reluctantly. "I'll be right down."

Driving down the hill, I go through my usual jumble of irrational emotions. First I'm angry at Elsa for having her fever, then irritated with Mary for not having called me earlier in the evening, and finally annoyed with Ginger for not waiting until morning. I'm glad I have this ride; otherwise I'd offend a lot of people. By the time I get to the nursing home, my irritation has subsided, and compassion for Mrs. Toivonen has begun to take over. Ginger is waiting for me in the dark hall just outside Mrs. Toivonen's room, chart in hand. "She looks pretty sick, David."

She does indeed! Wasted away to sixty-nine pounds, chronic bedsores on the bony protuberances of back and hip, she peers at me from behind her blank face. I'm used to all that from my regular monthly visits, but this morning there is no movement of her eyes, no resistance to my examination, nothing to indicate she's really there. Worse yet, there is little more to learn about the history of her fever than what Ginger has already told me over the phone. Mrs. Toivonen, of course, hasn't talked in three years, nor has she understood anything I've said as far as I can tell; so there is no hope of further information from her. My exam is brief as I look pointedly for the most common causes of fever in the elderly—upper respiratory infection, pneumonia, bladder infection, a viral illness. I realize I'm not being thorough, and feel briefly guilty as I recall an article I've read suggesting that nursing-home patients receive less thorough medical attention simply because they are old and feeble. It's true, of course. I know perfectly well that if this were a forty-seven-year-old schoolteacher in the emergency room with a fever, I would be spending an hour checking him out and talking with him. I try to assuage my guilt with the thought that I can't exhaust myself now, in the middle of the night, if I'm going to give decent care to all the other patients who need me in the morning. In my heart, though, I know it's a lousy excuse.

Listening to Mrs. Toivonen's chest, I hear the noises I expected, faint crackling pops indicating irritation in the lungs, probably pneumonia. I complete the rest of the exam without finding anything else and look up at Ginger. "I think she's got pneumonia," I say, and we both stare at Elsa's withered body. I wonder to myself, "What am I going to do now?" Ginger's glance tells me the same question is going through her head. I ask her to call Mark out of bed for a chest x-ray, and I write orders for a urine culture in the morning just to make sure a bladder infection is not causing the fever. While waiting for the x-ray, Ginger and I sit at the nurse's station, writing our respective reports in the chart.

Ginger looks up. "Mabel Lundberg said she hoped there wouldn't be any heroics if Elsa got sick again."

"I know. She talked to me, too." What does she mean by "heroics," though? I suddenly feel irritated again, but I keep my mouth shut; Almost thirty years younger than Elsa, Mabel is the only friend Mrs. Toivonen has, her only visitor at the nursing home. Mabel was a neighbor, and before Elsa's stroke she would help her with shopping, drive her to her clinic visits, run errands, and generally help out. She probably knows better than anyone what Elsa would really want, but Elsa's only relative, a niece I've never met who lives in another state, called some months ago asking that "everything possible" be done for her aunt. "Heroics"—"everything possible": each phrase refers to the same intervention but means something entirely different. We all want "everything possible" done for our poor, bedridden aunt; but at the same time we all want to spare her those terrible medical "heroics" in which doctors "prolong needlessly the agony of the dying." It all depends on the words you choose.

Essentially alone in the middle of the night, foggy from tiredness, I'll make decisions that will probably mean life or death for this old woman. I think back to medical school and university hospital where a thousand dollars' worth of laboratory and x-ray studies would have been done to make sure she really did have pneumonia: several x-rays of the chest, urine cultures, blood cultures, microscopic examinations of her phlegm (which could only be obtained by putting a needle through the neck and into the trachea of this sixty-nine-pound, eighty-three-year-old lady), blood counts, a Mantoux test to make sure she doesn't have tuberculosis, possibly even lung scans to check for blood clots. The list is limited only by one's imagination, each test "reasonable" in its own way once you enter the labyrinth of medical thoroughness. I can almost hear the residents suggesting obscure possibilities to demonstrate their erudition. (And are they wrong? Can any price be put on human life? Is any distance too far to go to discover a rare, potentially fatal, but curable illness?)

There in the middle of the night I consider doing "everything possible" for Mrs. Toivonen: transfer to the hospital, IVS for hydration, large doses of penicillin, thorough lab and x-ray evaluation, twice-daily rounds to be sure she is recovering, other more toxic antibiotics to cover the chance of an infection resistant to penicillin, even transfer to our regional hospital for specialist evaluation and care. None of it is unreasonable, and another night I might choose just such a course; but tonight my human sympathies lie with Mrs. Toivonen and what I perceive as her desire to die. Perhaps it is because Ginger is working, and I know how impatient she is with technological "heroics." Perhaps it is because I've been feeling a little depressed myself in the last few days and imagine I can better appreciate Mrs. Toivonen's perspective, although who knows what thoughts are—or aren't—going on behind the impenetrable mask of that face? Perhaps, I think to myself, it is because I'm tired and lazy and don't want to bother.

In any event, I decide against the "heroics," but I can't just do nothing, either. Everything in my training and background pulls against that course, so there is no way I'm going to be able to be consistent and just go home. Instead, I compromise and write an order in the chart instructing the nursing staff to administer liquid penicillin by mouth, encourage fluid intake, and make an appointment with my office so I can re-examine Mrs. Toivonen in thirty-six hours. My orders make no real medical sense, of course. Such a debilitated lady's pneumonia will probably require the higher doses of penicillin possible only through an IV; Mrs. Toivonen is also likely to refuse the nurses' attempts to give her extra fluids. And my compromise makes even less ethical sense. Am I or am I not treating Mrs. Toivonen? Am I or am I not prolonging her life artificially?

On my way out of the dark hospital, I talk with Mark, who looks sleepier than I feel, and we check the x-ray. I've known all along that the information it can offer me will be questionable at best. With her severe back curvature, Mrs. Toivonen is always difficult to x-ray, and she has chronic changes in her lungs which make early pneumonia difficult to detect. I thank Mark for the x-ray, wondering why I ever ordered it. Driving up the hill, I wonder why the practice of medicine is so often dissatisfying.

As usual, it takes me an hour to get back to sleep.

Mrs. Toivonen survived her pneumonia, more because of her constitution than my treatment, but even my compromise treatment was an important ethical choice. I had decided that the quality of her life was not valuable enough to warrant aggressive medical treatment. Situations like Mrs. Toivonen's are common. In my own practice and in those of other physicians I see around me, the old, chronically ill, debilitated, or mentally impaired do not receive the same level of aggressive medical evaluation and treatment as do the young, acutely ill, and mentally normal. Two physicians studied the response of a nursing-home staff to fevers in their elderly residents and discovered that the older and more debilitated the patients were, the less likely they were to receive aggressive treatment.[10] The nursing aide was less likely to bring a fever to the attention of the supervising nurse, the nurse less likely to call the physician, the physician less likely to examine the patient personally, and the fever less likely to be treated with antibiotics. During my student years I was working with a particularly caring and competent doctor. When the nurses one day on hospital rounds reported that a debilitated elderly patient had a fever, I was shocked to watch my preceptor write an order for aspirin without even investigating the cause of the fever. Without further explanation he lamely apologized to me by explaining that it was "probably just a virus." Only years later did I understand that this physician had developed his own way of allowing certain patients to die by withholding all available care.

Some may believe I acted irresponsibly and unethically in not treating Mrs. Toivonen more aggressively. There has been a widespread perception in medical circles that all patients should receive the maximum possible care for any given medical problem. In medical schools, in conversations between physicians, and—until very recently—in the medical literature, there has been the tacit assumption that all patients (with the possible exception of the terminally ill) receive the maximum care. But it isn't so. We rarely discuss this reality or debate its ethics. Only recently has there been acknowledgment that this extraordinarily common, profoundly disturbing ethical deliberation is a daily part of our lives. Instead, the practicing physician has been left to fly by the seat of his pants.

Some might be tempted to dismiss the entire problem with the simple assertion that all patients deserve maximal care. Consider, however, the following situation. We have in our nursing home a young woman who has been comatose for five years as a result of an accident. Although there is no meaningful chance that she will ever improve, she is not "brain-dead" and is supported only by routine nursing care, consisting of tube feedings, regular turnings, urinary catheters, and good hygiene; she is on no respirator or other machine. If, on a routine yearly examination, her physician were somehow to discover that she was in danger of a life-threatening heart attack within the next few years, few persons, I think, would recommend full-scale evaluation for possibly coronary bypass surgery. The decision not to offer her maximal care might be justified in any one of several ways, but most often the question would simply not arise. It would seem obvious to the practicing physician that this particular patient should not receive such heroic treatment.

I think few would quarrel with the decision to withhold such evaluation and treatment. But once we have allowed that some persons should not receive some treatments that will prolong their lives, we must begin the thorny ethical process of "drawing lines": which patients? which treatments? If this comatose young woman should not get the bypass surgery, then what kinds of treatment might we offer her? How far should we go? Would we perform a major abdominal operation to repair a dangerous ballooning of the aorta, a major artery that would otherwise probably rupture and kill her within a matter of weeks? Would we perform routine surgery to cure appendicitis? Would we give her an IV to compensate for fluid loss if she had diarrhea? Would we give her medicines by mouth to treat an uncomplicated urinary-tract infection? Would we put in a new stomach tube so that she could continue being fed? Each person might draw the line differently, but once it is agreed that a certain heroic treatment will not be offered, that still doesn't tell us what to do.

Because of his technical expertise (and his prestige in our society), the physician ordinarily also inherits the responsibility and the power to make such basic decisions about the value of a human life. The good and compassionate physician will, I believe, try to include the patient and the family in such important deliberations, but the physicians ability to phrase options, stress information, and present his own advice allows him enormous power in determining the nature of the care given. This power becomes, for all practical purposes, absolute when he is dealing with incapacitated patients, especially if family members are far away or otherwise not closely involved.

One might expect that the physician would have some special training or at least some resources to which he might turn when such common problems arise. But aside from his experience, no special training exists, and until very recently, almost no practical resources were available. There certainly has been a great deal published about the termination of life-support measures in persons whose brains are dead, but that problem is both simple and uncommon compared to a situation like Mrs. Toivonen's; the difficulties there are not so much ethical as technical—that is, how one determines for sure that the patient's brain is dead.

There has also been much discussion about care of the terminally ill cancer patient, but that situation is also much more clear-cut than the usual one of the debilitated elderly patient. The cancer patient and her physician can know that the illness will end in death within a certain period of time; therefore, the physician can reassure himself that he is not so much withholding available treatment as "allowing the person to die with dignity." (The professional ethicist may see little distinction between the patient terminally ill with lung cancer and Mrs. Toivonen, but the certainty of the former's death within a very short time compared with the possibility of Mrs. Toivonen's living for years creates an important distinction for the practicing physician.) Also, the relatively rapid course of terminal cancer allows the patient to know, while she is still completely lucid, that the illness is terminal. She can thus participate fully in the discussion of the matter before the decisions are made.

Charlotte Stroh was a sixty-three-year-old woman I had known well for several years when she first noticed the abdominal pain which eventually led to a diagnosis of cancer of the pancreas. After the diagnosis was established, Charlotte had a thorough discussion with the cancer specialist in Duluth. Although he offered her chemotherapy; he told her that it was unlikely to help very much and that there was almost no chance of a cure. Charlotte decided against any such attempts at treatment, since the side effects would probably make her very sick and prevent her from enjoying the last months of her life. She returned home with the intention of living as fully as she could during whatever time she had left.

At our next visit, Charlotte and I discussed her situation. She knew she had only a few months to live, and she knew she wanted to spend as little of that time as possible in the hospital. She was afraid not so much of dying as of the pain that might accompany the process. She wanted to be kept as comfortable as possible, but once she was really sick she didn't want anything to prolong her dying. If possible, she wanted to stay at home.

The terminal phase of her illness came quickly. We saw each other every two weeks, but she had dwindled from her usual 140 pounds to 110 within six weeks, and had become very jaundiced since the cancer was beginning to block the bile duct. Two weeks later she was confined to bed and beginning to have periods of delirium. There was not too much pain, and it could be controlled by regular shots of morphine, which her husband learned to administer. During the last days of her illness she developed a fever, probably as a result of an infection in the bile duct. It would have been possible temporarily to treat the infection or even surgically to bypass the blocked bile duct, but the question had already been settled. Charlotte had made it very clear how she wanted to die; besides, the heroic treatments would have added little to the length of her life and nothing to the quality. Charlotte died quietly at home.

Although much energy has been devoted to the ethics of treating the terminally ill and defining the meaning of brain death, the much more common situation of the elderly, debilitated patient who contracts an acute illness has been left relatively unaddressed. Ethicists, though, have advanced several helpful suggestions. Some recommend that the physician

sit down with his patient to discuss, in advance, what the patient might like
to have done under certain circumstances. Others suggest a "living will"
that would direct the physician to a particular course of action if the patient
became disabled. Perhaps the best course—now legally possible in many
states—would be to discuss the situation with a friend or family member
and appoint him or her "surrogate decision-maker" in the event the patient
becomes incompetent. Although these are helpful ideas, they have some
serious drawbacks.

First of all, few persons in our society want to think seriously about their
aging and death. Apart from offhand comments ("I hope they don't let me
linger on like that!"), most people do not want to confront the eventual loss
of their powers. Few are likely to make out a living will or pay their
physician for the privilege of discussing the possibility of their own
incapacity.

Secondly, a patient who has discussed all this with her personal
physician may very well be attended by someone else when these issues
finally arise. Not only do we live in an increasingly mobile society in which
the long-term physician-patient relationship is less common, but the very
structure of medical care almost assures a stranger for a physician when the
patient becomes seriously ill. Medicine has been broken down into minute
specialties. Even hospitals are organized according to the level of
specialized care available, from the local community hospital to the regional
hospital to the large university center. Patients, especially the very ill, are
handed from doctor to doctor, sometimes being attended by many at once,
and may even be transferred from hospital to hospital. The patient may
never have had an opportunity to discuss with the physician or physicians
who will attend her how she would like to be treated at the end of her life.

Furthermore, people's ideas about the quality of life change drastically
as they age, especially in the last years of their lives. The twenty-one-year-
old who would rather be shot than suffer the imagined ignominy of a
nursing home may be only too grateful to accept a nursing-home bed and
warm meals when she turns eighty-five. A living will or a frank
conversation with one's physician even at age fifty-five rarely would reflect
what one's wishes will be at age seventy.

Martin Hooker was not atypical. At ninety years of age, his heart failure
kept him very sedentary. With much help from friends and family, he had
managed to remain living at home. Yet he was often short of breath and
weak, and required frequent hospitalization to rest and have his medications
adjusted—his "tune-ups," he would call them. Finally, he developed a
disease in the heart's natural pacemaker which, while not aggravating his

heart condition, could have stopped his heart at any moment, causing sudden death. I explained the situation to him and outlined his choices. Without hesitation, he chose to travel to Duluth and have an artificial pacemaker inserted surgically. Life for him, despite his severe limitations, was still very valuable. Months later Mr. Hooker developed abdominal pain and yellow skin, which suggested a cancer in his liver, gall bladder, or pancreas. When our preliminary tests in the hospital indicated that he probably did have cancer, Mr. Hooker chose not to have any further evaluation or treatment, and he died within a few weeks. Although I did not know him when he was younger, I doubt whether he could have predicted his decisions even fifteen years earlier.

Most important of all, it is simply too difficult to define in advance all the varieties of illness, suffering, prognosis, and treatment with sufficient precision for the definitions to be much help in the actual situation. A physician may know, for instance, that a patient does not want to be "kept alive unnecessarily if I'm a vegetable and there is no hope of improvement." Unfortunately, the real-life situation will almost surely be much more complex. What constitutes "keeping a person alive"? Is it giving her a warm room and regular meals rather than allowing her to lie at home alone, paralyzed, and with no heat? Is it giving her an IV or routine antibiotics? And what quality of life constitutes "being a vegetable"? Furthermore, in real life there is rarely any certainty about prognosis. Improvement may be unlikely, but it is often possible. So even in the best case in which a self-aware person has talked with her physician or made out a recent living will, the complexities of the actual situation probably will render those efforts of little practical use to the physician, and because of her debilities or the seriousness of her acute illness, the patient herself is rarely fully available to her physician at the needed moment.

Although any of these suggestions would be of some benefit to the physician in deciding how aggressively to treat an elderly, debilitated, and incompetent patient, very few patients actually make any such preparations, and the physician is thrown back on his own judgment. Since he does not know what the patient would in fact want, he cannot make what the ethicists call a "substituted judgment" for the patient and must act instead in the patient's best interest. What the ethicists mean by "best interest" is that the physician should take into account everything about the patient: relief of suffering, preservation of functioning, quality and extent of life, and the impact of the incapacity on loved ones' lives—surely an impossible task for one doctor in the middle of the night.

If the professional ethicists have not yet provided much help in this most difficult situation, the law has been positively confusing. As I understand it, some recent court decisions have suggested that the court must authorize the withholding of treatment in any particular case. Although I would not argue with the attempt to relieve the physician of this responsibility, the facts are that these decisions usually need to be made quickly (within hours or days), repeatedly (quality of life, prognosis, and treatment options may vary from day to day), and with a considerable degree of medical expertise. It is unrealistic to believe that the courts could decide these matters promptly even if we decided they should. It will be interesting to see how the courts finally settle the issue, but I expect physicians will get little help, regardless.

In fact, then, I, as the primary care physician, face this complex dilemma alone. I may try to share the decision with the family, who may know how the patient would decide in such a situation, but most often they have even less idea of what to do than I and are desperately relying on me for guidance. Even when someone in the family does have a definite idea of what should be done, the situation is hardly less murky for the physician. Although our society may believe that a patient has the right to refuse treatment, we do not indiscriminately assign that right to any relative who might think he knows what is best.

I first met Maria Alvarez when her regular doctor, my partner, had to be out of town for the week and I began seeing her at the hospital. Before my partner left, he told me some of the details of her case. Although she was only thirty-eight, Maria was dying of a rare and very malignant stomach cancer. Abused as a child, she was full of anger, which she found it difficult to express appropriately, a situation aggravated by her terminal illness. She had never married, had no family in this country, and had few friends. After she became ill, an older friend, Guadalupe Adriano, began taking care of her and eventually invited Maria into her home as Maria became too weak to care for herself. Maria was also befriended by an order of Roman Catholic nuns for whom she had previously worked as a domestic. They visited her daily whenever she was in the hospital. According to my partner, Maria had chosen to refuse the radiation therapy that might have prolonged her life because she was ready to die and didn't want to suffer the nausea that the radiation often produces. As her only "family," Guadalupe had been part of the decision too. Both she and the sisters felt that Maria had already suffered enough, and they supported Maria's decision to decline the potentially life-sustaining treatment.

Maria had been in the hospital about a week when I first saw her. She was obviously very weak, had lost a great deal of weight, and had to be totally cared for by the nurses. Her English was poor, so Guadalupe was there that first Friday to translate for us. I introduced myself and asked her how things were going. Through Guadalupe, Maria told me she was still having a lot of pain in her stomach but the morphine shots made her fairly comfortable; she complained, however, that the nurses wouldn't give her the shots often enough. I told her I would check to see how often the shots were being given. I then asked about the radiation treatment.

"Dr. Peters tells me that you've decided against having the x-ray treatment to your stomach."

"Oh, yes, Doctor," Guadalupe answered without translating. "Maria and the sisters and I have talked about it many times. Maria has suffered so very much. There is no need to make it go on longer."

"Well, could you ask Maria now, just to be sure, if she is still certain that she doesn't want it?"

Guadalupe and Maria talked for a minute in Spanish, and Maria shook her head weakly and said, "No, Doctor, no x-rays." I nodded my head, we chatted for a while together, and I left.

Guadalupe was out of town for the next few days, so Maria and I had to get along on our own. Although I had difficulty talking with her each morning as I made rounds, I sensed that the language barrier was not the only problem. Maria was withdrawn but also seemed angry. I couldn't get her to talk about what was bothering her, so I asked Maryanne Doherty, Maria's nurse, how she behaved the rest of the day. Maryanne said that Maria was uncomfortable but communicative. She had been asking questions about the radiation therapy the entire weekend. I walked back to Maria's room.

"Maria, Maryanne said that you have been asking about the x-ray treatment."

Maria looked quickly at me, her eyes flashing with anger. "Doctor, why you not want me to have x-ray? I having much pain. Maryanne say x-ray help stomach pain."

"Who told you I don't want you to have the x-ray treatment, Maria? Guadalupe said you didn't want it. It might be a good idea, and it might help your pain."

"Guadalupe say you doctors think x-rays not good for me. X-rays make me sick. X-rays not help. But Maryanne say x-rays make pain better."

"We don't know for sure, Maria. The x-rays will probably help your stomach pain, but they may make you nauseated...sick to your stomach. I'll help you decide, but it's your decision, not mine."

It was difficult to talk together since Maria was obviously still angry with me and not sure she could trust me. As I deciphered her story, I began to understand. Guadalupe and the sisters had seen Maria in such pain and discomfort that they had evidently decided palliative radiation treatment was not in her best interest. Since Guadalupe was Maria's main source of medical information, she had—unconsciously, I suspect—slanted that information against the radiation treatment. Until Maria was left alone with the nurses for the weekend, she had believed that everyone was advising her against—no, essentially refusing her—the radiation therapy. Surrounded by the uniform opinions of Guadalupe and the sisters, Maria didn't want the therapy, but when left alone in the hospital to face her illness, she decided she did.

Our language barrier and the absence of a family made Maria's situation different from the usual debilitated elderly patient's, but what it does illustrate is that often the closest and most well-intentioned person is precisely the one who has the most difficulty in knowing what the patient wants. Guadalupe was undoubtedly not purposely distorting Maria's wishes; she was simply grieving deeply for her friend's pain and could not bear the thought of potentially life-prolonging treatment. Maria, of course, was still competent to make a decision by herself; but if she had become suddenly incompetent, Guadalupe—apparently an ideal surrogate decision-maker—would have been leading me astray. For better or for worse, then, the decision invariably comes back to me, if only to evaluate the objectivity of the surrogate decision-maker.

It is not that I believe I should be making these incredibly important decisions about life and death by myself. The fact is simply that under our current system of medical care, I do. So what do I do, then? Medicine has developed no rational way to make such decisions about which treatment to give and which to withhold once heroics have been ruled out. Perhaps my most frequent response land I do not admit this easily is not to make a conscious decision at all. Aware that Mrs. Toivonen has a fever, I may decide to see her at the end of office hours and then, in the rush of the late afternoon, "forget" to drop by the nursing home until the next morning, by which time she is either getting better or is so much worse that "it won't help to put her in the hospital anyway"; or if I do examine her promptly, my examination will not be so thorough as it might be, and I will decide that the fever is "only a virus" when I really haven't excluded all the likely possibilities; or, as I did this time, I will give some treatment that will probably help but is not as aggressive as it could be.

The problem is simply too painful for me as a single human being to face day after day in a conscious way. How do I decide to let this person die when everything in my being says that life is the ultimate value? How can I make a decision about the quality of someone else's life without even knowing what she would want? On the other hand, how can I inflict the pain of aggressive treatment, impose the suffering of further living, and spend scarce resources of time and money on this life that is so obviously trying to end itself? Since I am operating in a vacuum and have no reliable criteria with which to make a judgment, my choice is ultimately guided by my feelings, prejudices, and mood more than by my reason. Occasionally, feeling the burden of this decision-making to be heavier than usual, I'll turn to a partner, if time and circumstances allow, and discuss the situation. Almost invariably she or he will agree that my proposed course of action "seems reasonable," which is reassuring and of some help emotionally. However, the value of such agreement between two people of the same age, training, vocation, economic status, and social position (who, in addition, are professionally constrained from directly criticizing each other) is questionable at best.

Although I made these sorts of decisions quite routinely for seven years, the cumulative emotional impact was severe. The underlying irrationality of the judgments gnawed at me; the life-and-death importance of my actions kept me awake at night; and the guilt and depression of never really knowing whether I had acted properly wore away at me; for I knew I was being forced into decisions that only God should make.

Physicians are often accused of harboring a God complex and of being defensive about their decision-making. I would like to suggest that, at least in this circumstance, we have been forced into a godlike role. What other choice now exists? If challenged, many physicians would undoubtedly launch into a passionately logical defense of whatever particular ethical decisions they tend to make in such cases. I can easily understand such reactions. Trained to act in everything with impeccable logic and rationality, physicians naturally find it hard to look at the underlying irrationality of whatever they do in these situations, and such defensiveness is a very understandable emotional reaction to having to make ultimate decisions for which there are no criteria.

■

A few years after trying to decide whether or not to treat Mrs. Toivonen, I wrote about my experience in the *New England Journal of Medicine*. In reply, I received more than one hundred letters—almost all from doctors— several articles, and one full-length book dealing with the subject of decision-making for the "incompetent" patient. The thrust of the letters, the articles, and the book was that although such decision-making is difficult, it is not impossible and there are established ethical principles for almost all conceivable situations. In fairness, neither the articles nor the book had been published when I was wrestling with my conscience, but my reading simplified the matter for me somewhat and gave me some guidelines for my own future work. In fact, because of my article I became something of an "instant expert" and was asked several times to speak about the issue.

As I gave these talks on medical ethics to other physicians, however, I realized that figuring out ethical principles played only a small part in learning how to deal with the stresses of difficult ethical decisions. From the distance of the speaker's platform, it was easy enough to suggest that all patients have the right to refuse treatment, that a living will can guide the physician, that the physician can make decisions about treatment with the next of kin, and so on ad nauseam. Retrospectively, such principles frequently seem quite clear. In real life, however, one is not only confronted with the specific ethical dilemma of what to do with Mrs. Toivonen, but also faced with exhaustion from the intensity of one's daily work, burnout from the need to be constantly available, strain from the overwhelming knowledge needed to deal with even her limited condition, uncertainty as to her diagnosis and prognosis, awareness of the mistakes one has made in similar situations in the past, and concern that one spend public money wisely. Indeed, even ethical expertise may only become one more field of specialized knowledge that chides one's ignorance.

Presenting these stresses for analysis one at a time, then, oversimplifies the problem. The practicing physician confronts them not only simultaneously but also on the run, when he is tired, alone, and hurried. He does not have the leisure to mull a problem over and deal with it from a considered perspective. He is continually making decisions while emotionally and physically on edge.

Nevertheless, physicians do deal with these stresses. We have found ways to continue practicing in the face of this pressure. How do we respond? The language we use hints at the answer. We begin by learning to detach ourselves from the chaos of the situation. Mr. Smith with all his fears and insecurities becomes "the stroke in room 8," thus allowing us to concentrate on his physical disability; Mrs. Jones, who regularly disrupts the office with her incessant demands, becomes "a problem patient" whom we manage with behavior modification. We next learn the principles of efficiency and productivity. "Patient management" is the buzz word, and "productivity incentives" are standard practice at many large clinics to encourage greater efficiency in office and hospital. Then the physician discovers the protective coat of prestige and authority. When I told Mrs. Murphy that we had done everything we could to treat her husband's cardiac arrest, I was using the power of my position to close off questions, to protect myself from her implied criticisms. Any continued questioning would have been a direct challenge to me, a step only the most assertive sort of person might take. In addition, we physicians protect ourselves emotionally by keeping ourselves at the top of the medical hierarchy. How often is the physician "Dr. Hilfiker" while the nurse is "Maryanne"? Finally—though no language hints at this—there is our wealth to comfort us. If we must suffer outrageous stress, at least, so the unspoken theory goes, we will be well compensated financially.

These responses—clinical detachment, efficiency and productivity, prestige and authority, hierarchy, and wealth—are not intrinsic to the practice of medicine. Although the structure of modern medical practice may encourage them, we physicians also choose to endorse and accept them, in part as a way to relieve the inordinate pressure of our work. They seem to offer a kind of escape. Unfortunately, the escape is only illusory. Let us look at them one by one.

Chapter 9

CLINICAL DETACHMENT

"DAVID! IT'S HAPPENING...NOW! There's blood all over the place! I'm scared. What should I do?"

The panic-stricken voice on the other end of the phone is Margaret Laine's. Thirty-two years old, a professional in the community, Margaret possessed an independence and energy that had earned her a special place in my affection. I was pleased she'd selected me for her doctor when she suspected her first pregnancy. During our initial interview I was surprised by her nervousness and anxiety concerning the pregnancy. I suppose I had unrealistically assumed that her outwardly calm and urbane manner reflected an imperturbable inner self. Nevertheless, our initial visit was filled with the usual good feelings of early pregnancy.

During our second visit, however, I was unable to hear the baby's heartbeat, which by then should have been audible. Although I feared an impending miscarriage, I couldn't be sure and didn't voice my concern to Margaret; but I was not surprised when she called me a few days later to report small amounts of vaginal bleeding and some abdominal cramping. She came in for another exam, and this time her pregnancy test was negative. It was clear Margaret was in the process of a miscarriage. She was upset, of course, but we reviewed in some detail the possible causes of the problem and what might still happen, and I instructed her in caring for herself until it was over. Since most miscarriages will complete themselves without medical intervention, there seemed no need for any special treatment.

"David? What should I do? Am I bleeding to death?"

Almost reflexively, I respond to Margaret's panic with a deliberate calmness. "Tell me what's happening. You're bleeding vaginally?"

"Yes! What should I do? There's so much blood."

"When did you start to bleed so heavily?"

"Just ten or fifteen minutes ago. I had some cramping and then a big gush of blood. I'm still bleeding...a lot!"

I consider for a moment sending the ambulance, but a corner of my mind reminds me that since most people have so little experience estimating blood loss they tend to exaggerate greatly the amount they're losing. "I think this is what we talked about in the office, Margaret. You're probably getting rid of the fetus right now. Have Mark bring you down to the emergency room immediately, and I'll meet you there."

Ordinarily, I wait for the emergency-room nurse to phone and tell me that the patient has arrived before I leave home; it's amazing how long it can sometimes take even an "emergency" to travel the few blocks to the hospital. This Sunday morning, however, I remember Margaret's previous anxieties and her frightened voice just now and decide to meet her at the hospital door. I drive down immediately. Even so, Mark is there ahead of me, already helping his wife into the emergency room when I arrive. But Susan Metcalf, the head nurse for the shift, pulls me aside before I can get into the room.

"Dr. Hilfiker? Charles is having trouble in room 4. He seems to be having some kind of a seizure. I called you at home, but your wife said you'd already left."

"Charles?" For a second I don't connect, then I remember: Charles Lind, forty-four years old. I admitted him ten days ago with severe constipation and was very much surprised to diagnose cancer of the large intestine. He went down to Duluth, of course, but returned yesterday: inoperable cancer with no significant treatment available. Although seemingly still in his usual health, Charles had come home to die. I admitted him to our hospital again for a few days of rest before he went home, with no expectations of immediate complications. "What happened?" I ask Susan, trying to sort out priorities between Margaret and Charles.

"He was just finishing lunch when the seizure started. He's coming out of it now, breathing regularly, pulse normal, and he didn't hurt himself, but he's unconscious."

I look at Margaret through the open door, and she looks back at me imploringly. What do I do now, attend to her or Charles? Automatically, my mind moves into that detached consciousness I know so well. I separate myself emotionally from the situation, trying to ignore for a moment Margaret's panic, Susan's concern, even my own feelings. I must make myself stand aside, observe it all from a "neutral" and "objective" point of view, make the best decision possible. I know Margaret's scared, but from the way she looks and is acting I think she'll be all right for a few minutes. I have no idea what's really happening to Charles. "Susan, please stay here with Margaret, and make sure she's all right. I'll check on Charles." I turn and call through the open door, "Margaret, someone is having trouble over at the hospital. Susan will stay with you, and I'll be right back." I turn and leave before she has a chance to reply.

Whatever Charles's problem is, it's almost over by the time I get to his room. The nurse's aide is holding his head, and his eyes are still rolling, but he soon relaxes and drops off to sleep. I examine him quickly, but there are no obvious problems now. The aide describes what was probably a seizure, for which there is no obvious immediate treatment, so, still in that emotionally detached frame of mind, I ask the aide to stay with Charles while I return to the emergency room.

Margaret is almost hysterical. "David, I think I'm going to die. Please help me. I'm so scared."

Her fear is only too understandable. She's been grieving over the loss of her baby, and now these torrents of blood, more than she's ever seen before, shift her concern to her own death. Once again I feel the privilege that allows me behind the masks people wear, the privilege to be with Margaret in her fright and confusion; but I can't allow myself to stay with those feelings for Margaret until I'm sure she's physically safe. I remain in my clinically detached state of mind: "What's her blood pressure, Susan?"

"A hundred and thirty over eighty."

An adequate blood pressure. I ask Margaret some technical questions about her bleeding: When did it start? Can she estimate more precisely how much bleeding there has been? Has she passed any tissue? Examining her, I find the dead fetus wedged in the cervix. No wonder she's still bleeding! I grasp the tissue with a forceps and easily pull it out. There is a gush of blood, which quickly slows down to a trickle. I examine her uterus to find it contracted and hard. Good! It's over.

I begin to relax a bit and return from my place of emotional separation. Despite Margaret's sorrow and anxiety, I almost look forward to the next part of the process: describing to her with some confidence what has happened, reassuring her, sharing her grief. But a voice over the loudspeaker interrupts me: "Code Blue, room 4; Code Blue, room 4."

"Excuse me, Margaret. You're going to be all right. I'll be back as soon as I can." I run out the door, sensing the anger underneath her fear. Of course, she understands that I have to leave, but that won't do much to ameliorate her feelings of fear, her feelings of anger for receiving such fragmented care when she most needs attention. As I run for room 4, I hope Susan will stay with Margaret. Margaret needs her substantial expertise more than I do.

Rushing into Charles's room, I find the two aides have begun cardiopulmonary resuscitation on Charles. One looks up at me while she continues to push rhythmically on Charles's chest. "He's had another one, David. Then he stopped breathing entirely, and we couldn't find a pulse. We started CPR right away."

Once again, by strong force of habit, I am already far away from my emotions and the bustle in the room. What's going on? This is obviously no simple seizure. Charles has no history of heart attack or stroke. Is this somehow related to his cancer? I'm not sure of the underlying cause, so I begin to deal with the situation as it is: no heartbeat, no spontaneous breathing, Charles's pupils already unresponsive to a light shined into them. While continuing to do CPR, we hook up the heart monitor: a straight line—no heartbeat. It doesn't take me long to resolve the ethical problem. There seems no reason even to attempt a prolonged resuscitation only to deliver Charles to a lingering death by colon cancer. I'm not sure what caused his sudden death—probably a heart attack or a stroke—but nature seems to have saved him considerable suffering. I stop the resuscitation efforts and ask the aide to call Charles's family.

As I return to the emergency room, I can feel my emotions beginning to roil. Clinical detachment works very well for its intended purpose— allowing me to function as precisely as possible as a medical technician in emotionally turbulent waters—but the necessary suppression of feelings leaves me agitated and exhausted. Susan has indeed stayed in the emergency room, but Margaret is still wild-eyed when I return. The bleeding has slowed considerably, and I'm confident the worst is over; however, despite what has been a real closeness in our relationship, Margaret doesn't seem to trust my assessment of the situation: "There's so much blood, David. I feel like I'm going to die."

I admit Margaret into the hospital for observation, examine her thoroughly to detect any unforeseen problems, and spend considerable time with her trying to explain and comfort. It is not an easy task, but it seems well worth the time spent. Finally, I leave Margaret in Susan's care and turn to Charles's family to try to explain to them as much as I can of what happened to him.

When I arrive home, my emotions are a tangled web. Laurel, my oldest daughter, wants to show me her Sunday school project, but I can barely muster the patience. I go outside and begin to work on the woodpile. It feels good to lift the heavy splitting maul and slam it down, sending the birch pieces flying. The physical exertion begins to bring the parts of my soul together again. Only then does the nagging doubt begin. Should I have terminated the CPR so quickly on Charles? Was there anything else we could have done to resuscitate him? Would he have wanted an extra month of life to say farewell to his family and friends even if it would have meant a more painful death? I work for several hours before I can even face my family.

Separating oneself from the immediacy—the panic, fear, anger, desperation, confusion—of a situation is probably a necessary device the physician uses as protection from the emotional consequences of medical practice. Indeed, this clinical detachment is essential to certain aspects of that practice. The emergency situation, for instance, calls for swift, exact decision-making. Temporarily, at least, the situation needs to be objectified; decisions need to be analyzed and determined logically; the person must become a "patient" whom one treats according to previously learned principles. The physician's own fear of what is happening, the patient's fears, the physician's likes and dislikes, must all be shunted aside temporarily (or perhaps, treated as one more complicating factor in the decision) in order to give the patient or patients the best possible care.

Such detachment is requisite in more routine patient encounters as well. The recent explosion of medical knowledge has armed the physician with considerable knowledge, precise diagnostic tools, and a substantial therapeutic armamentarium. The physician has to be intimately acquainted with a vast quantity of information and technically competent in a variety of procedures. In dealing with even the most routine medical diagnostic problem, the physician must remember each of the myriad of technical questions that should be asked in the interview. She must select the appropriate type of examination for the illness. She has to requisition from hundreds of possibilities the proper laboratory and x-ray tests. Most important, she must sift through all the information obtained and, if possible, establish a diagnosis and a treatment plan.

To perform these technical tasks adequately, the physician must detach herself from her own desires, hopes, and fears as well as the patients wishes and emotions. The patient's desire for a particular diagnosis, a particular method of testing, or a particular treatment must not be allowed to interfere with the physician's learning about the disease; although the patient's desires should become paramount later on, when a decision must be made about treatment (a shift that, as we shall see, is not always an easy one).

Thus, a primary role of the good physician is that of scientific technician, and the scientific attitude is one of detachment. (It is still hoped, of course, that the physician will remain a warm human being, a good counselor, an empathic person; but without the technological skills and attitudes of a scientist, the physician of today simply cannot do her job.) Although the physician may care deeply about the patient as a person, she may be required, during a significant portion of her contact with that patient, to ignore the person and concentrate on the disease.

Not surprisingly, the physician, under the pressures of everyday doctoring, often begins to use this tool of clinical detachment for another purpose: as personal protection. By objectifying the stresses of medical practice, treating them as further scientific problems, the physician seems to spare herself their consequences, to protect herself from burning out. By defining herself as an objective scientific technician rather than as a servant, and by replacing messy emotions with scientific detachment the physician can even deflect the call to constant availability. What begins as a necessary tool in certain areas of medicine easily becomes a generalized defensive response.

The unintended consequence is that the person tends to disappear and the patient becomes an object, a thing upon which the physician acts. It is no accident that the talk of medical personnel is filled with references to people as if they were diseases or parts of the body. "Dr. Hilfiker, there's a broken leg in the ER" may sound humorous out of context, but it reflects the reality of medical detachment.

Once this temporary period of detachment is over, it would, of course, be desirable for the physician to shift back into the role of caring counselor, noticing and attending to the patient's emotions, responding with feeling to the patient's needs. (Indeed, in deciding which of a series of options for treatment should be chosen, the patient's needs should be a key consideration.) But I did not find this shifting back and forth so easy to regulate, for detachment became not only a necessary and useful perspective for disease evaluation but also a comfortable place to stay. After a while, it came to seem that my efficiency and productivity depended upon my ability to detach myself. My power resided in my technical abilities. Compared with such power and efficiency, the imprecision and give-and-take inherent in the empathetic relationship often appeared inefficient and irrational.

Amanda Blake is a sixty-five-year-old woman I had not known until her daughter, Rebecca Dahlquist, dragged her into the office last week. Mrs. Blake had had a poor appetite and had been losing weight for several months before she agreed to see the doctor. Rebecca had called me previously to explain that her mother had a drinking problem and always refused to come to the clinic even for routine examinations. Aside from the poor appetite, the weight loss, and a little bit of stomach pain, I found nothing. She wouldn't talk about her drinking, saying that it was Rebecca who drank too much and I should talk to her. I ordered some routine tests and asked her to come back in a week to discuss the results. I was surprised two days later when the blood tests showed some damage to the liver and an elevation of the bilirubin level suggesting an obstruction of the bile duct. I called Mrs. Blake and asked her to go over to the hospital for an ultrasound picture of the abdomen when the visiting radiologist came up from Duluth. Sure enough, the pictures showed what was probably a tumor in the pancreas.

I'm half an hour late for Mrs. Blake's appointment and really haven't taken the time to prepare. Worse yet, I already know it's going to be difficult. Pressed for time, I plunge right in without even finding out how the suspense and worry of the last week has affected Mrs. Blake. I don't even take the time for the usual pleasantries that might make her feel more comfortable.

"Mrs. Blake, I'm worried about the results of your tests. It looks like there's something blocking the bile duct coming from your liver. Some liver enzymes were elevated in your blood, and your pictures yesterday showed something in the pancreas which is probably blocking the duct. I think we'd better have a specialist in Duluth examine you and get some more tests to find out what's going on."

"Dr. Hilfiker, you don't mean I have to go down to Duluth for an appointment? I don't know if I can leave Earl for a whole day. He's not feeling well himself, you know."

"I'm afraid one day won't be enough. You'll need to be in the hospital so the specialist can do the necessary tests; they may even need to do an operation to find out for sure what's wrong."

"Oh, Doctor, I can't do that. Who will take care of Earl? Besides, I don't think I'm that sick. I'll just try to eat a little more and maybe it'll get better."

I don't know whether Mrs. Blake simply doesn't understand the potential seriousness of her situation, is denying the problem altogether, or is simply frightened out of her wits by what I'm saying; but I can feel my impatience rising. "Mrs. Blake," I say, my voice sharp with irritation, "the pictures show a tumor in the pancreas. I don't think—"

"A tumor! My mother had a tumor and my sister just died from a breast cancer. It was awful!" She begins to cry.

"Mrs. Blake, we don't know for sure this is a cancer," I say evasively. I don't want to deal with her tears or her fears or her denial right now. I want to get her down to Duluth where a definitive diagnosis can be made. "The tests just show something blocking the bile duct. That's why I want you to go to a specialist—to find out what's really wrong."

"Can't you take care of me up here? Couldn't I just wait until spring when the roads are a little better? You know how slippery they are now. I don't think Earl could drive me all the way down."

Some part of me is aware that we are no longer talking about an appointment in Duluth but are deep inside Mrs. Blake's emotional response to her illness. I know I should slow down and be present for her as she experiences her feelings, but I don't. I press on.

"I don't know for sure what's wrong, but you have to go down to Duluth right away to find out. You've waited a long time already to come in," I say, regretting the words as soon as they are out of my mouth. The last thing she needs right now is to feel guilty about not having taken care of herself.

"Oh, I know. Rebecca wanted me to come in way last October, but I was afraid it might be cancer. I didn't want to come in. Oh, who will take care of Earl?"

"Maybe Rebecca could drive you down. I'll call Dr. Young to make an appointment for you."

"Dr. Young? Isn't he the cancer specialist? He took care of my sister. Then you do think it's cancer?"

"Mrs. Blake, I can't be sure yet." I stand up. "Dr. Young will be the best doctor to find out whether it's cancer or not. Is it OK if I call him?"

She nods her head, and I leave to make the phone call.

On the way back to the examining room, I realize I've blown it. It only took me a few minutes to review Mrs. Blake's laboratory and ultrasound results, assimilate it into her previous history, and know that she needed referral. A wiser part of me knew it was going to take much longer to deal with Mrs. Blake's emotional and spiritual response to my findings. But I just didn't want to get into it, so I tried to stay in the security of my technological expertise instead of entering the murky world of her fears and dreams. Rather than spend the time and energy necessary to sort through her conflicting priorities, her confusion, her fear of death, I found it only too tempting simply to insist that she see the cancer specialist. I stop for a moment in the hallway and take a few deep breaths. "Marge, please tell whoever's waiting that I'll be a while. I have to spend some more time with Mrs. Blake. See if some of the others could reschedule."

Living in a culture that values efficiency and productivity, I suppose it was only natural for me to want to avoid the confusion of Mrs. Blake's world. My increasing unwillingness to empathize as fully as possible with my patients never represented a sudden change, nor was it ever complete. Frequently, as with Mrs. Blake, I would catch myself and move from my place of detachment into a more feeling relationship; but gradually I found myself residing more and more in my slightly detached, objective form of consciousness, away from the overwhelmingly painful stresses of real life.

It was simply too emotionally wrenching to be constantly bounced back and forth between detachment and involvement. The two forms of consciousness were so different, in a sense so contradictory, that the tension between them became difficult to sustain. It might have been obvious from an objective point of view that Mrs. Blake needed further technological evaluation; but immersion in her swirling world of fears and dependencies, values and feelings, might have revealed the unsuspected conclusion that she would indeed be happier, that her life would be better, without drastic technological intervention to discover a cancer that would probably be incurable anyway.

The conflict became too great, not perhaps the first time I made the shift, but the 1,458th time I had to go back and forth between my rational, objective, technological world and the imprecise fluidity of the physician-patient relationship. To make matters worse, my growing sense of detachment began to carry over into my personal life. I became so accustomed to the rationality and clarity of professional aloofness that I began to expect my family, my friends, and my colleagues to operate out of the same clear consciousness.

To give but one example: Karin, our middle child, had frequent stomach aches as a part of minor illnesses or as a response to stress. Marja would tell me as I walked in from the clinic about Karin's latest stomach ache, and I would wearily climb up into the loft to examine yet another "patient." The diagnosis was usually obvious, and I would tell her that I didn't think it was serious and that it would probably go away in a little while. I would then climb down and eat the supper that Marja had saved for me. Only infrequently did I remember that Karin did not so much need a doctor as she needed a father. She did not so much need a diagnosis as she needed someone to comfort and reassure her, to go get the hot-water bottle, to talk with her about which of her problems might be causing the stomach ache.

I had always been a rational, logical thinker; my emotional and intuitive side had always been underdeveloped—unfortunately true for many physicians; but the clinical detachment so necessary to medicine exacerbated such tendencies, encouraging me to emphasize them. Slowly, over the years, the habit of dissociation became so ingrained in my personality that it invaded every nook and cranny of my life. I simply expected all of us to live that way as a matter of course. It wasn't that I consciously valued that attitude toward life; but so powerful was its attraction, so difficult was it to switch out of it, that I found myself living with it more and more. What had begun as a technological tool became over the years a dominating force in my life.

Chapter 10

EFFICIENCY

"YOU'RE GOING TO NEED your track shoes this afternoon," Jackie says as I walk into the office.

Glancing at the overcrowded schedule, I cringe. The morning was hectic and I've just returned from our semi-monthly hospital medical staff meeting, scheduled over lunch hour so as not to waste any time. Now it looks like I'll need to hurry through the afternoon, too.

My first patient is Bill Martin, who needs an insurance physical. As I enter the examining room, he's sitting on the exam table, undressed except for his shorts. He hands me his papers. I glance at them and notice he hasn't filled out his medical history. "Didn't Marge have you fill out these forms?" I ask impatiently.

"No, I, uh, just got here, I guess. I thought you were supposed to do that."

He's right. Most insurance companies want the physician personally to ask the twenty-five or so routine questions and fill in the answers in the examining room; but it seems like such a waste of time, especially on a busy office day, that Marge usually asks my patients to fill out the forms while they are waiting. I then review the answers briefly in the examining room. It seems like a reasonable shortcut.

I consider handing the form back to Bill to fill out, but realize I have no one else to see right now since he's my first patient of the afternoon, so I resign myself to the inefficiency. Over the next ten minutes Bill tells me that, no, he hasn't had recent surgery, rheumatic fever, malaria, or gonorrhea; that his parents died at seventy-two and sixty-seven of heart disease; that he's not sure when his last tetanus shot was. I feel somewhat foolish interviewing Bill without his clothes on, but I certainly don't want to waste more time in the examining room while he dresses and undresses.

By the time we complete the interview and examination, I'm already fifteen minutes behind schedule, and the afternoon is just beginning. My next patient, sixteen-year-old Terra Sims, injured her wrist a few minutes ago doing gymnastics over at school. After a brief examination, I send her to the hospital for an x-ray. Marge already has little Stacie Montgomery ready in room 2 for a re-check of her recent ear infection; but Stacie needs a hearing test first, so I ask Marge to perform the audiogram while I turn my attention to Ray Dunder's abdominal pain, which has been bothering him for the past several weeks. It's a complicated problem. After a thorough history and physical, I send him over to the hospital for some blood tests. At the same time, Marge is just putting Bob Morgan into the minor surgery room with a hand he lacerated while cleaning fish. Stacie is waiting in room 1 with her hearing test; Terra is back from the hospital with her x-ray. I check Bob's hand to make sure it needs suturing and ask Marge to get him ready while I look at Terra's x-ray. It turns out she has cracked a bone in her wrist and will need a cast. I send her over to the hospital emergency room (where we do all our casting) to have the nurses there get the supplies ready while I talk to Stacie and her mother about her hearing.

The afternoon crunch is beginning: a lacerated hand in the minor surgery room, a broken wrist in the emergency room, abdominal pain cooking in the laboratory, patients backed up in the waiting room. There is no possibility of taking things one at a time, of finishing one before beginning another. My patients will be spread out over two buildings in various stages of evaluation until the last person returns from the lab at five-thirty this afternoon.

The purpose of all this confusion is to use my day "efficiently." Since my time is almost the only thing patients pay for in our clinic, it must be used well in order to cover clinic expenses and salaries. It is considered important that every minute be spent as productively as possible. The office routine is consequently arranged so that I can see the maximum number of patients in the shortest possible time.

Much is written in the mountain of throwaway journals, paid for by pharmaceutical ads and distributed free of charge to physicians, concerning "modernizing" or "streamlining" patient care. "Time management" is big business in medicine, too. How many examining rooms should one doctor have available for efficient use of his time? Four rooms is not unusual. How many nurses should work with one physician so that the office runs smoothly? At least one, and often two or even three. How can routine tasks be performed in advance so as not to waste office time? What tasks can the nurse perform so the doctor can be more efficient? Physicians often talk about "productivity," about "patient management," for ours is a business.

Our clinic physicians tended to resist this pressure to become maximally efficient. We never approached the productivity we heard about from our colleagues in other clinics. Nevertheless, the ideal of efficiency had a definite effect on our practice patterns, as it must on those of all physicians. It was important, for instance, to have patients waiting in several different examining rooms at the same time. I could not afford to wait for a patient to fill out a form, take a hearing test, have blood drawn for laboratory work, have an x-ray, or be made ready to have a laceration repaired. It was not at all unusual to be evaluating five or six patients almost simultaneously. It did not even seem particularly difficult. I would simply store away in different parts of my brain information concerning different patients and recall it when necessary. I was surprised how seldom the information got confused. (It was one of my partners who, late one night during his internship training, finally returned to seventy-three-year-old Mrs. Johnson's room to tell her sleepily that he had determined her symptoms were caused by an early pregnancy!) So as not to waste any time, a new patient had always to be ready in an examining room in case I finished the previous appointment early.

I felt I should not interrupt my interview and examination to wait for patients to undress for the examination. The nurse, therefore, determined the general nature of the problem in advance and had each patient appropriately disrobed before I came into the room. The demand for efficiency dominated, even though it often meant long interviews with only a sheet for protection, even though I knew from my training that patients would not talk as freely when interviewed undressed. In fact, I practically convinced myself that a state of undress helped patients "get to the point" more quickly.

A tight schedule seemed necessary for maximum efficiency; and there was always the temptation to schedule even more heavily just to make sure a patient who required less time than expected would not leave me with nothing to do. The tightness of this schedule, in turn, hurried me along. One tends to be more efficient when one is an hour behind schedule.

All other staff members had to organize their jobs so that I could be maximally efficient. Nurses had to spend long periods doing essentially nothing to be sure they were ready to help me exactly when I needed it. They also had to do as much as possible to prepare the patient for her exam: take vital signs, get the forms filled out, perform various tests, set up for procedures—all so that the physician would not have to waste time on "nonessentials." In many clinics, nurses or assistants do a major portion of the interviewing, handle most phone calls, take care of some medical problems completely on their own. There is nothing inherently wrong with this, of course, if the nurse is trained to handle these functions; my point is that the purpose of these adaptations is usually only to increase the physician's productivity. Since the salaries of nurses and other office personnel were so much lower than ours, it "made sense" to have them do as much as possible to allow us to concentrate on the tasks that only we could do.

The drive for efficiency and productivity around which modern medicine is increasingly structured derives in large part from the physician's busyness. Having too much to do seems an integral part of the physician's life from medical school on. There is always more to learn in medical school than can possibly be assimilated, more to do in internship and residency training than can possibly be done in twenty-four-hour days, more problems to take care of as a practicing physician than can reasonably be accommodated. It seems only natural to look for ways to streamline the process.

Another major force behind efficiency and productivity is money; for a physician's charges are not so much structured around the amount of time spent with a patient (although this is a factor) as around the procedure performed. I will probably charge you the same amount for taking care of your sore throat in five minutes as I would if it took me ten minutes. The "complete history and physical examination" that takes me only twenty minutes because the patient is young with no significant problems and has filled out her history form in advance will probably be billed at a rate as high or almost as high as the history and physical of an older patient with many more problems which takes me forty minutes. Thus, my efficiency in "processing" my patients in less time means more money per hour.

Even beyond these two more or less practical factors of busyness and money, efficiency and productivity seem to have acquired a sort of independent life and value all their own in the world of doctoring. In our training the surgeon who could perform an appendectomy in twenty minutes rather than forty became, in our minds, the better surgeon; the intern who could keep up with the steady flow of patients into the emergency room came to seem better than the slower, perhaps more careful one. Thus efficiency and productivity became a yardstick for measuring oneself as a competent physician.

On a different level, the perceived need to be efficient and productive gave us as physicians a large measure of control over others. The rest of the office staff clearly had to structure itself to maintain the doctor's highest efficiency. Routine tasks could always be passed along to one of the office staff on the grounds of making the doctor's time more efficient. Syringing wax from young children's ears, for instance, was an unpleasant and difficult task, since the children frequently became frightened and irritable. Even though I could usually do the procedure more quickly and less traumatically (my hands, bigger and stronger, more easily manipulated the large syringe, and I was skilled with some fine tools for working within the ear canal to remove especially resistant bits of hard wax), I usually passed on the task to Marge since it would "save so much of my time." I also passed on as much paperwork as possible to Marge and the other staff members. All of this made sense, of course, but it also served to cement the hierarchy, to place me firmly in control. Patients, too, could be manipulated by my need to be efficient. Practically any interchange could be cut short on the basis of busyness. All I had to do was stand up, and patients knew they had only a little time left. Even outside the office in a small town that valued social involvement, I was rarely asked to volunteer my time to various causes. It was assumed I was too busy. Thus, to a certain extent, efficiency and productivity became goals because they allowed me to set my own agenda over the needs of others. When the doctor's highest efficiency becomes a primary value, the doctor sits atop the hierarchy: everything works for him. From there it is only a short—if improper—step to the assumption that the doctor is per se superior, more valuable.

In the medical profession's discussion of efficiency and productivity, it is of course assumed that these values do not compromise the care offered to patients. To read the articles in the journals of medical economics, one would believe that adding an extra examining room (and keeping one more patient waiting) so the doctor doesn't waste any time has no negative effects on the quality of care; one would believe that using a form to secure a history allows an equally good (or even better!) history to be taken, that having patients wait undressed in the examining room does not interfere with good medicine. Borrowing from the corporate model, the quality of the work is judged primarily by its immediate technical results. As long as we reach the correct diagnosis and prescribe the right treatment, then shortening the process as much as possible seems to be an excellent goal.

What is overlooked is the side effects on physicians, nurses, medical technicians, clerical staff, and patients. There can be no question, of course, that some measure of efficiency is required. The days when the doctor personally sat down with the patient and performed everything from registration to laboratory tests are gone—if they ever existed. Specialization of function is simply a fact of our era, and there can be no question that many physicians could make changes in their day-to-day behavior which would allow them to see more patients in less time without significantly compromising the care they render. But there can also be no question that there is a trade-off. Although I may be able to diagnose a child's ear infection and write a prescription to treat it within ninety seconds, it does not follow that it is good medical care to do so. I may cure the ear infection without ever having dealt with the mother's questions about what caused it, what to expect over the next several days, or what to watch out for in the future. I have not established any relationship with the child that will encourage her to see me as someone toward whom to turn for help in the future. I have not allowed relaxed time for the mother to ask her "Oh, by the way…" question which may be as important to her as her daughter's illness. I have cured an earache. All else remains undone.

Meredith Heasley brings her two youngest boys to the office one day in early spring. Both eight-month-old Robby and two-year-old Jason have colds, replete with green snot draining constantly from their noses and deep coughs. Meredith is a close friend, and I'm a little surprised she's brought the kids to the clinic; it's a long drive from their homestead, and the Heasleys generally pride themselves on their home remedies and independence from my office. I examine the boys and mentally start tape number 43, "Reassurance To Mothers Whose Young Children Have Colds." But Meredith isn't listening. I look more closely, and her eyes are glistening. I stop in mid-sentence and just wait. In the silence the tears come gushing forth.

"I'm so sick of these colds, David. The boys are sick all the time, whining and crying. John is gone most of the day and I'm cooped up inside the house. I can't even go for a walk without dragging the boys with me. I feel like I'm going to crack up. First there was the pregnancy and then my bad back. My back's still aching and I'm constantly worn out. Nobody comes to visit, and it's too far into town to drag the boys all the time. That little cabin we've got seemed so romantic three years ago, but I can't stand it any more. I'm going crazy!"

I encourage Meredith to tell me more, and she talks for nearly fifteen minutes without interruption. Difficulties in being straightforward with John, cabin fever from the long winter, having to lay aside many of her personal goals to rear the children, spiritual struggles she can talk with no one about, Meredith is bursting with conflicting feelings. I listen, I remind her of other mothers who felt like they were going crazy when their children were young, and we explore possibilities for resolving some of the tension. What began as a routine fifteen-minute appointment to evaluate colds has developed into something much more important. It would not have happened had I taken care of the presenting problems more efficiently.

In medical school classes on interviewing technique, the importance of open-ended questions is stressed. Such questions as "How have things been going for you?" or "How can I help you?" encourage people to expand upon their needs, to talk about what is important to them at the time, which is crucial if one really wants to discover as much as possible about a patient's physical and emotional state. Open-ended questions are not, however, very efficient. It is much quicker to ask whether a patient has pain anywhere or has a fever than to give her a chance to talk about whatever is on her mind. After all, the patient may need to take a circuitous route to get to the real problem, a route which may bear no relationship to the fifteen minutes the schedule has allotted her. If I am concerned primarily with efficiency, I may never discover the nature of the problem that really concerns the patient.

Nor can a personal relationship between a patient and a physician be accomplished efficiently. It takes time. Fear of illness, concern about medications, and distrust of the physician cannot be handled efficiently either. Indeed, a concern with productivity discourages dealing with these problems at all, since the patient may come to think that they are not important enough to make it onto the agenda. A major concern with efficiency inevitably leaves the impression of busyness. Most patients simply will not or cannot share many kinds of problems without a relaxed and open atmosphere.

There is also the intimidation factor. The doctor leads the interview, examination, and explanation of results. The patient's anxious questions—her real concerns—flee her mind as she tries to fit into this smoothly running machine; and if one of her questions does occur to her before she leaves the examination room, she may hesitate to ask it: it seems out of place. More than one patient has apologized to me for taking up my time with what turned out to be a very significant personal issue. If an atmosphere of efficiency and productivity makes it difficult for the patient to express her needs, this atmosphere is even more deleterious to the physician. As more and more emphasis is placed on the need to be productive, patients are increasingly seen as products, as objects to be moved through the clinic as quickly as possible, as things to be manipulated. Naturally enough, physicians then come to see themselves more and more as efficient machines processing products. "How can we move Mrs. Smith most efficiently through the office?" is not so different a question from "What kind of assembly line is best for making a Ford?" This reality was most effectively burned into my consciousness by a change in the method of computing our salaries which occurred during my last years in our clinic.

For the first five years of my practice, I received a regular salary with no incentives to encourage maximally efficient use of my time. Since the clinic was losing money, there were periodic exhortations from our clinic administrator to bring more income in, but there was no fundamental shift in the way we dealt with patients. About this time our clinic administration changed from a large, multiclinic corporation in a city far away to a local, community-owned clinic with an elected board of directors. Being persons of good business sense, our directors soon suggested that our personal income be proportional to our productivity. For every dollar we booked in patient charges in excess of what we had generated when we were on straight salary, we would receive a percentage of that dollar as a bonus. The more money we brought into the clinic, the more we would be paid. The idea seemed wonderful! No physician would be forced into greater efficiency than he desired, for the system would be voluntary, but there would be an opportunity to earn more money. And the clinic would gain, too, since a percentage of the extra dollars would come to the clinic. Everybody was satisfied.

The system worked beautifully. From the very first months it went into effect, each physician consistently booked more than he had when he was on salary. The clinic fared better financially; we dispensed with the periodic exhortations from the administrator; the physicians were satisfied. It seemed the perfect administrative step. And there were no drastic and terrible changes in physician behavior, either; personable, caring physicians did not suddenly turn into money-grubbing mercenaries. But gradually I became aware of a profound change in my own perception of my relationship to my patients. When old Mrs. Hilden came into the clinic to complain for the fortieth time about her nervousness and tired feet, I no longer had the same patience. I knew it was going to take me twenty or thirty minutes to listen to her sympathetically, suggest a few changes in her regimen, and leave her with the feeling that somebody cared. Yet I knew I'd only be able to charge her for a regular office call (which Medicare would discount), whereas I would be able to generate twice or three times as much income doing almost anything else.

I tried not to let it affect me, hated myself when I caught myself thinking about it, but there it was. Patients and their inconvenient questions, requests for explanations, or long-winded ways of presenting themselves became objects blocking productivity in the office. I found myself less interested in open-ended questions and more interested in surgical procedures (which are charged at a much higher rate). Gradually, as the idea of efficiency took hold, we physicians even noticed that it was harder to get together for our weekly journal club where we discussed recent professional articles. Our semi-monthly meetings to discuss problems of general concern with the public health nurses were now more and more frequently sacrificed to a procedure we had scheduled or to prolonged hospital rounds. We started holding physician meetings at 7:00 A.M. so as not to interfere with the daily schedule.

In the short term, the sacrifices were hardly even noticed. We did not immediately become worse doctors for missing our journal club meetings, and the public health nurses could still take care of our patients without our relaxed discussions together. The effects were hardly measurable; but in the long run having fewer meetings together isolated us from one another, gave us less opportunity to share new ideas. Medical misconceptions that I had somehow acquired had less chance of exposure to my partners' knowledge; new bits of information took longer to become disseminated. Because the public health nurse and I had not coordinated our messages, I sometimes found her recommending rest to a patient when I was recommending activity. Our 7:00 A.M. meetings caused longer days and grumpier physicians. Not infrequently, one of us, having been up on call much of the previous night, would fail to show up for an especially important 7:00 A.M. meeting, leaving the rest of us disgruntled at the wasted time. Our practices became more individualistic and insular as we had less contact with one another. Efficiency has its price.

As with clinical detachment, then, the attempt to respond to the pressures of medicine by becoming more efficient inevitably damages both the physician-patient relationship and the physician's own concept of self. Yet the issue is a subtle one. It is simply not possible to refuse to consider the demands to be productive and efficient, for they are important issues in our task of caring for patients—especially since physicians are still in short supply. Yet these values have such a profound effect on the practice of medicine that the physician needs to remain constantly aware of the trade-off between efficiency and deeper personal relationship, between productivity and medicine as an art. When the physician finds that he is not taking the needed time for reflective meditation upon the meaning of his job, when he finds he is using laboratory tests and x-ray studies instead of in-depth interviews, when he is giving pills instead of counseling or explanation, when he himself is not getting his needed sleep: at these points the physician needs to ask himself whether the values of efficiency and productivity have not in fact gained the upper hand, submerging other important medical and human values. Has productivity become a goal in itself? Has the attempt to meet more and more patient needs ultimately turned into its opposite? Has the physician become a servant, not of his patients, but of productivity and efficiency themselves?

Chapter 11

AUTHORITY

"DOCTOR, I'M FORTY-FOUR years old, my kids have all left home, my husband is all wrapped up in this new job of his, and I'm a nervous wreck."

Betty Darcy has come to my office this morning for the express purpose of obtaining a prescription for Valium. She sits awkwardly on the examination table, fully clothed, clutching her purse. She seems surprised and irritated by my reluctance to write her the prescription she wants.

"I'd go to see that marriage counselor you suggested, but my husband isn't interested and besides talking isn't going to help anything. I've been nervous all my life. My whole family is nervous. When we lived in St. Louis, my doctor always gave me Valium. It really calms me down when I need it. I don't know what I'll do if you won't give it to me."

I take a deep breath. This is not my favorite way to start the day. I don't have much to offer Mrs. Darcy. We live in a crazy-making society where loneliness, alienation, social pressures, and affluence have created an entire subculture of people struggling to cope. The counseling I've suggested probably wouldn't help her since she seems less interested in fundamental personal change than in simply feeling better. Almost hopelessly I wonder how I am going to communicate to her a perception of tranquilizers that is so different from her own.

Stress, anxiety, insomnia—emotional disease is the developed world's major epidemic. It infects us all, and each of us, at some time or other, probably yearns for "something to calm me down a little." The symptoms are for many people so overwhelmingly distressing that in the 1950s the introduction of minor tranquilizers (Valium, Librium, and so on) to alleviate some of the suffering was hailed as another of medicine's modern miracles. The pills seemed to help. Valium and the others became the most widely prescribed drugs in the country. It took considerable experience, much reflection upon the nature of societal illness, a deeper understanding of the nature of drug addiction, and indeed, a basic change in the physician's perception of her responsibility to her patients to convince many of us that the use of tranquilizers should be sharply curtailed. Over time, we came to believe that the minor tranquilizers should be used only infrequently, temporarily, and under strict control. Not all physicians have come to this same conclusion. Certainly our society as a whole has not come to a consensus on the matter. Thus, Mrs. Darcy and I face each other over a gulf that has as much to do with values as it does with strict medical judgment.

She knows that the Valium makes her feel better. She is not a drug addict in the sense that she lies around all day staring at the ceiling in a drug-induced high. She has used tranquilizers for years without, in her mind, experiencing significant side effects. She really doesn't understand why I won't write her a prescription.

I believe with equal fervor that the Valium does not enhance her quality of life. My belief is born of my observations of other patients and nurtured by my personal experience that one improves only by confronting the source of one's loneliness, alienation, and anxiety. The good feeling that the tranquilizers provide, the "cure" for the anxiety, will not change the underlying causes of Mrs. Darcy's problems. The symptoms would only be masked, taking away (at least temporarily) any need to pursue the underlying difficulty. Is it better to live with one's head pleasantly clouded by tranquilizers or to face the suffering of one's life and make the requisite changes? It is not, of course, an equal contest, this value struggle between Mrs. Darcy and me, because I have the ultimate power, the power to refuse to write her a prescription, and there's not much she can do about it. She wants her Valium, and I don't want to give it to her, and that's that.

To make our morning confrontation emotionally more difficult for both of us, Mrs. Darcy will end up paying my office the usual $17.00 charge (plus a $5.50 fee to open a new chart) for the opportunity to be told that I will not write her a prescription. During our fruitless fifteen-minute conversation I am, strictly speaking, her employee, yet I am—for no reason understandable to her—refusing her request for a prescription. It is little wonder she perceives me as arbitrary, authoritarian, and insensitive, or that I leave the consultation feeling alienated from her.

As I sit next to the exam room in the closet-sized dictating booth, trying to decide what to put in Mrs. Darcy's chart, I realize at least part of the reason patients so often perceive physicians as authoritarian, why the consultative aspect of the relationship is so frequently lost. We physicians are given numerous legal and social responsibilities—many of them largely unknown to our patients—which are frequently in conflict with the patient's goals and desires. We are also given the authority to pursue these responsibilities. Without some doctor's permission in the form of a prescription, for instance, Mrs. Darcy cannot get her tranquilizer. This morning she is not interested in my expertise or my advice; she needs me as a "ticket" to get what she wants. I, on the other hand, have the legal responsibility to see that prescription medications are used wisely and correctly. (The fact that there are often no precise guidelines for "wise" or "correct" usage only exacerbates the situation, forcing me to rely on my own values, not necessarily any less arbitrary than Mrs. Darcy's.) That patients must pay me for this act of social responsibility further complicates the situation.

To a major degree this conflict is inevitable, since the physician frequently acts as an agent of society against the desires of the patient. When one also takes into account the physician's institutional authority (to regulate medications, to admit to the hospital, to order laboratory and x-ray evaluation, to authorize absences from work, and so on), virtually every patient encounter places the physician, in one way or another, in the role of granting or denying patient desires. For better or for worse, the physician is not simply a consultant to the patient, an employee in his service, but also society's gatekeeper, with considerable power.

A physician's authority, however, is much broader than the legal power she possesses; for the physician is usually allowed to define reality and to make judgments about meaning and value that her patients will have to accept as valid. The physician's study of science, her understanding of the causes and treatment of disease, and her position of respect within the community allow her to tell the patient what is wrong with him and what he should do. To the extent that patients accept that authority, physicians can define the causes of stomach pain as a stressful life-style, can judge psychotherapy more valuable than tranquilizers, can make cost/benefit judgments that are essentially value judgments—though none of these is, strictly speaking, a scientific conclusion. As a physician, then, I have not only legal or social authority but also a cultural authority that is largely unquestioned. Unfortunately, once one gets used to such an ego-gratifying position, the fine line between appropriate and inappropriate use of this power becomes all too easy to cross.

Mark Siipola comes to see me an hour or so after Mrs. Darcy leaves.

Thirty-two years old, a Vietnam veteran with a lame foot, Mark is a burly, vigorous man. I've been treating his bouts of migraine headaches for some years, but this morning he has a different complaint.

"Doc, I've been feelin' real tired lately. It seems like I got no energy or drive or anything. Even my wife noticed it. As soon as I come home from work, I lie down in front of the TV and go to sleep. Something's got to be wrong. This just ain't like me."

Tiredness is one of the more frequent patient complaints and one of the more difficult for the physician to deal with. Even with a relatively thorough evaluation, I will usually not discover a specific cause for the complaint. Nevertheless, possible causes are many and can prove important. From cancer to anxiety, from anemia to marriage problems, virtually any illness or emotional distrubance can present itself initially as tiredness. In fact, tiredness is not so much a symptom as the perception that "something is wrong with me." Despite the frequent failure to pinpoint a cause for tiredness, the physician must evaluate the patient's entire health status to deal adequately with the complaint.

Our interview yields some clues but nothing definite. Mark is overweight. He's also under considerable pressure at work, and there is stress in the marriage. He's smoking two packs of cigarettes a day; his migraines have been worse lately; and he has a family history of heart disease and cancer. However, aside from his obesity and a slightly elevated blood pressure, nothing shows up from his physical. Since Mark is very much concerned about his symptoms and disinclined to believe they are due simply to stress, overweight, and smoking, I order the routine blood cell count, blood chemistry profile, thyroid function tests, urinalysis, and chest x-ray. Three days later, when Mark returns for a review of what has been discovered, all the tests and the x-ray have been reported as normal.

"Doc, there's *got* to be something wrong. I just don't feel right. Yeah, I know about the weight and the cigarettes, but that's been the same for ten years. This can't all be from stress."

I can't be certain, either, that his symptoms are from stress, although that seems the most likely possibility. What I don't tell Mark is that there are countless more laboratory and x-ray tests that could be performed to look for obscure causes of his tiredness: x-rays of the stomach and intestines; x-rays of the kidneys; special hormonal studies to rule out rare causes of disease whose first symptom might be tiredness; blood cultures to look for silent infection. The likelihood of any of these tests providing useful information in this situation is minuscule; moreover, they are expensive, any one of them costing more than the entire office interview and examination.

My opinion that these specialized tests should not be ordered in Mark's situation has been shaped by my training, by my years of taking care of similar problems, by my belief that serious disease would soon declare itself in specific symptoms anyway, and by my own rough attempts to perform a cost/benefit analysis. Ultimately, however, such an analysis is based on values that may be different for Mark and me. I have concluded that it is not justifiable to spend this amount of time and money trying to nail down with absolute certainty the etiology of certain symptoms when I can be relatively certain they come from stress.

This is not, however, a decision-making process I share with Mark. Although it seems proper that he participate, although he would pay for the tests himself (leaving me with no formal institutional responsibility), I find the prospect of trying to share this complex decision with him too time-consuming to consider on such a busy morning. Each test has its own probability of detecting various diseases, and this probability depends on what other tests have been ordered. Each disease has its own probability of being present, which influences the utility of each test. Each test has its own technical uncertainties, making it more or less reliable. Patients vary tremendously in their ability to understand these intricacies even when I take the time and effort to explain. To complicate matters further, my charges to Mark (upwards of a dollar a minute) mean that any attempt to include him in the process will generate even more expense for him.

More significantly, I have become accustomed to assuming the authority of such decision-making. If the issue seemed more important, I might take the time and energy to explain all the various possibilities, but it just doesn't seem worthwhile this morning. So I compromise and explain to Mark that we have ruled out all the likely causes of tiredness and that his symptoms are probably due to the stresses of his job and his marriage. I suggest that if the attempt to reduce his stresses doesn't alleviate his symptoms, I could then investigate more intensively or refer him to a specialist. In this oblique way, I feel I've given Mark the opportunity to press for a more intensive examination now if he so desires—although I know perfectly well that he won't and that all I've really done is assuage my own guilt over not sharing these decisions with him.

As a new physician fresh from my internship, I was amazed at the considerable authority invested in me, not only in my consulting rooms but also among office and hospital staff and even within the general community. My patients to a large extent obeyed me, the staff deferred to my decisions, the community respected my opinions even in nonmedical matters. My position as physician automatically conferred upon me an authority that was independent of my abilities.

Indeed, some patients seemed to experience a relief in turning over their responsibility to me. The middle-aged vacationer admitted to the coronary care unit with his first heart attack might be chief executive officer of a large corporation in Minneapolis, but in this situation of stress and fear he needs to turn his authority over to someone who knows, or seems to know, what is going on. He does not want to debate possible therapies I might offer and their respective side effects; he wants me to make the decisions, to make them rapidly and well, to make him better. In that situation, of course, it may be appropriate to accept the authority, to reassure him that he is in good hands, to be the expert who—by his simple presence— comforts.

But I soon discovered another facet of the issue: how much protection that prestige and authority could give me. If the intensity of the job and the constant demand for my availability left me too tired, I could simply refuse a request for an explanation by implying that I had no time. No one would question me. If I was uncertain about a patient's diagnosis or about my competence to perform a certain procedure, I could feign confidence. Few would challenge me. If I made a mistake, I could ignore it. People would rarely call it to my attention. If I felt unsure about an ethical decision, I could do what seemed best to me. My authority protected me from scrutiny. My position of prestige became an oasis in which I could shelter myself from the stresses of my work.

My authority, then, began as something thrust upon me by the nature of my work. It seemed unavoidable, a part of the job. As time went on, though, I noticed myself using that authority even when it wasn't necessary. Despite its disadvantages, authority seemed a convenient tool.

As it turned out, the authoritarian relationship created as many problems as it solved. First of all, responsibility for the patient's health came to rest completely on me, while the patient remained passive, waiting to be cured by my magic incantations. Rather than take responsibility for his own health and well-being, the patient continued to see himself as a helpless victim, thus neglecting to bring his full powers into the recuperative process. At the same time, since medicine is an uncertain science in which mistakes happen, in which cause and effect are often unclear, the entire burden of this uncertainty fell on me when I did not share the decision-making with my patients. It was an overwhelming burden to take on alone.

After Maiya Martinen had gone to Duluth for her ultrasound examination because her fetus seemed small, the obstetrician who examined her called me, and we decided together that she could safely be delivered in our local hospital. I informed Maiya of our decision and the reasons for it, but I did not really offer her the option of delivering in Duluth with all the potential advantages of a large center. After Marko was born and had his first seizure in the delivery room, I diagnosed the seizure as due to low blood sugar and did not recommend that Marko be evaluated immediately by the neonatologist. Once again I made that decision by myself without including Maiya or her husband. I assumed—without really reasoning it all out—that the Martinens would have made the same decisions had I taken the time and effort to inform them fully, and so felt no need to go into all the details with them. It was a routine use of my authority.

When Marko's severe seizure disorder and brain damage finally manifested themselves, however, I felt the full weight of the responsibility I had so easily taken on. Those nagging and ultimately unanswerable questions about what might have caused the problem were mine to deal with, since I had made all the decisions. After it was all over, the Martinens never questioned me about those decisions (I suspect they were too intimidated by my position of authority), but they could not have helped but wonder. Anything that I could have said at that point would have had the clear ring of defensiveness. We found it, in fact, almost impossible to talk about the potential causes of Marko's disease.

Such an authoritarian relationship created a nearly impassable gulf between my patients and me. Since I was the expert, authority, decision-maker, the one to be obeyed, the relationship could not be an equal one. Whether the patient accepted it (thus legitimizing the distance between us) or fought against it (thus creating an adversarial situation), each of us was separated from the other, unable to solve our mutual problem. In addition, relationships of this sort gave me an exaggerated sense of my own importance. All day long I was being asked for advice. All day long I was considered indispensable. Even outside the office I was treated with deference. It was only too easy to perceive myself as inherently more important than others.

The prestige and authority that accompanied my position as physician seemed initially very attractive, almost adequate rewards in themselves for all the other pressures of the job. In the end, however, they helped to isolate me from the healing relationships with my patients that might have allowed me to handle the stresses of the job in a more balanced way over a longer period of time.

Chapter 12

HIERARCHY

IT IS EIGHT O'CLOCK in the evening of a very long day. This is the most intense rotation in the fourth year of medical school—internal medicine, six weeks of twelve-hour days and long nights. I am anxious to get home, but too tired to hurry. I sit wearily at the nurses' station desk, writing the results of the interview and examination on my last patient. Beside me Dr. Martin Oberdorfer scribbles some orders hastily in a chart and slides it toward a young nurse who is working on a chart of her own.

"Angie, make sure Mrs. Dimmerling in 702 gets that diet change right away," Dr. Oberdorfer says as he hurries down the hall.

The young nurse glares after the disappearing staff doctor. I know Dr. Oberdorfer only by reputation. Thirty-five years old, he's supposedly one of the best cardiologists on the university staff, but he's incredibly demanding. Students, interns, and residents all cringe before his frequently sarcastic reviews of their work-ups, and even other staff doctors are afraid of his sharp criticisms. He's known for his long days, his unfailing dedication to his patients, and his frequent harangues of errant nurses.

Angie (I don't even know her last name) lays her own work aside and starts to copy the orders for Mrs. Dimmerling. "Who the hell does he think he is?" she mutters to herself. "I can hardly read this." I continue to write, but I'm listening, almost without knowing it, to Angie's angry comments to herself.

"Beth," Angie says as she walks over to an older nurse on the other side of the nurses' station, "I can't even read this. What's Oberdorfer want here?"

"Hmm. I'm not sure. Looks like two teaspoons of Maalox every two hours."

"Yeah, I guess you're right. Two teaspoons. Wait a minute! Oberdorfer never orders two teaspoons of antacid. Remember him getting on that poor intern for not ordering enough. He said you always order at least two tablespoons. Remember him quoting that journal article about antacid efficacy? He can't have meant two teaspoons."

"Yeah, but he sure didn't write two tablespoons. That's got to be two teaspoons. Why don't you page him and ask?"

"Oh, sure, page Oberdorfer and tell him he blew it. 'Dr. Oberdorfer,'" Angie mimics herself in a singsong Southern drawl, "'I think you just made a mistake. You didn't really mean two teaspoons of Maalox, did you?' Come on, Beth, remember when Tricia tried to correct him? He just laid into her and ripped her apart. He wrote 'two teaspoons' and Mrs. Dimmerling's getting two teaspoons."

"I suppose so. It won't hurt Mrs. Dimmerling any, and maybe it'll teach Oberdorfer a lesson. I wouldn't count on that, though."

Angie and Beth return to their work, and I try to return to mine. I can hardly believe what I've just heard.

As I made my way through the years of medical training, I was often astounded by the rigidity of the medical hierarchy. Attending physicians were on top, followed by residents and interns. Even the residents had to be careful not to step on the toes of the attending physicians, but it was the gap between the physicians and the rest of the hospital staff that was the widest. Physicians made their evaluations and wrote their orders in almost complete isolation from the observations and opinions of the nurses who were in charge of the patients' care on a day-to-day basis; and physicians never even talked to the aides and orderlies, who had the most intimate and prolonged contact with patients. The only way physicians crossed the gap between themselves and the rest of the staff was by writing orders; it was very difficult for information to flow the other way. Hospital nurses, for instance, "chart on" each patient at least once a shift, describing that patient's status and what has been done for her; yet it was unusual indeed that a physician took the time to read the nurse's notes in the chart. Nurses would complain privately about a physician's behavior, but it was a rare day when they said something to his face.

We students were, so to speak, off to the side of the hierarchy, not really in the competition yet, so the nurses or aides would sometimes confide their resentments to us and express the hope that we would be different, that we would include them more as a part of a team. I learned during my internship that a nurse could be an invaluable ally in caring for a patient. On our obstetrics rotation, for instance, it almost seemed there was a testing period. For the first few days, the obstetric nurses watched us carefully to see whether we would include them. If we chose not to, they would simply perform their own jobs, very politely and competently, while we interns were left to stew in our own juices. In my own case, I knew I needed all the help I could get and went out of my way to consult the nurses as colleagues. For the rest of my rotation I was, almost literally, taken by the hand and instructed in the finer points of obstetric care. "Dr. Hilfiker, if you have the patient lie on her side, that fetal distress you're noticing may go away." "Dr. Hilfiker, you might want to put in the soft-tipped catheter for an IV rather than the steel needle; it stays in a lot better when she's moving about in labor." I even got advice about how to get along with my attending physicians: "Dr. Hilfiker, Dr. Adams doesn't like to be called too early on his patients; I think you can wait to call him about Mrs. Susnik."

Furthermore, nurses, both by training and experience, knew more about the meaning of illness within a patient's larger life. They were the ones who were usually around when patients would confide something important or when the family would visit. It was not unusual for the nurse (or the aide) to know that a patient's brother had died of a heart attack just before the patient's first episode of chest pain or that a patient who kept finding new physical complaints on the day of discharge was actually scared to return to her apartment alone.

Yet as I moved into practice, I discovered that the medical system had been so constructed as to keep the physician not only atop the hierarchy but also responsible for everyone else's performance. Nursing staff, pharmacists, physical and occupational therapists, laboratory and x-ray technicians, and public health nurses are all highly trained professionals, yet they can carry out many of their proper functions only with the authorization of a physician. A prescription is necessary for most drugs, as well as for physical therapy and occupational therapy. Written instructions in the chart are required for much nursing care provided in the hospital. Laboratory and x-ray tests are performed only with written instruction from the physician. From the legal point of view, the physician is responsible for the malpractice of other members of the health care team even if the error lies completely with the nurse or x-ray technician. Thus, the physician is encouraged to see himself as the leader of a team all of whose members are dependent upon him.

Such an organization may help promote efficient functioning, since some person has to take over-all responsibility for coordinating patient care, and the most appropriate person is often (though not always) the physician.

However, what may be a legitimate way of organizing a group of people can very quickly degenerate into authoritarianism. In medical jargon, physicians "order" a nurse to administer medications, implying a relationship between doctors and other staff members which may never be appropriate. Certainly, it leaves little room for the kind of cooperation that is basic to a supportive workplace or good medical care. (In addition, it's only a small step for the physician to start ordering his cup of coffee from the same nurse.)

Fifty-five-year-old Adela Jacobsen has been in the hospital for two weeks now with low back pain. All of her x-rays are normal, and there has been no sign that the nerves to the legs are being affected, so she would be a poor candidate for referral to a neurosurgeon. Ordinarily, a week or so of absolute bed rest with hot packs and massage applied to the back should improve things considerably, but Adela has not responded to the hospitalization at all. I listen to her bitter complaints again this morning, find nothing new on my examination, and leave the room to write orders at the nurses' station.

"I can't understand why she's not getting better," I say to Nancy Bjorkling, handing her the chart with new orders for extra hot packs and massage to be done by the nurses on every shift when the physical therapist is not available. Nancy has been on the nursing staff for a number of years, and we know each other well; the hard glint in her eyes tells me she's disturbed by something. "What's the matter?" I ask. "You look upset."

"Dr. Hilfiker, I don't mind giving patients whatever they need to help them get well, but Mrs. Jacobsen is treating this hospital like a hotel. She's on her buzzer every two minutes, and your orders have us giving her everything she wants. Most of the girls cant stand to be with her, she's so demanding. The only time she seems to have any back pain is in the morning when you come in. She bounces around the room like a sixteen-year-old the rest of the day. I don't think these extra massages are going to do anything except irritate the nurses on night shift."

"Oh," I stammer somewhat feebly. "When did all this begin?"

"We've been charting it practically every day for a week."

"Oh," I say again, stupidly, realizing I haven't bothered to read the nurses' notes in Mrs. Jacobsen's chart since she was admitted. "Why didn't somebody say something?"

"Well, you know, it doesn't seem right. But Mrs. Jacobsen's been too much. I think we're making her worse with all the attention we're paying her. She knows her back's got to stay sore or she gets kicked out of the hotel. She treats us like maids. Everybody's noticed it."

I'm embarrassed. Nancy and the others have understood Mrs. Jacobsen perfectly. The next morning I go into Mrs. Jacobsen's room to outline a plan of increasing ambulation; if she's not ready to go home in three days, I warn her, we'll have to transfer her to the nursing-home side. Two days later, she is sitting on the bed waiting for me during morning rounds, ready to go home, miraculously cured.

Many nurses now have four years of college education, including intense practical training, yet their ability to act independently is often sharply curtailed. In the midst of a busy evening of caring for a patient who has recently had a heart attack, chasing a senile patient down the hall, and coaching an unmarried mother through her first childbirth, a nurse will then have to track down a physician to authorize even an aspirin for a patient's headache. Nurses' skills are too often under-utilized, leaving them feeling frustrated and unfulfilled.

What we call each other is symbolic. Too often the physician remains "Dr. Hilfiker" long after the nurse has become "Annette." Physicians usually perceive themselves as bosses, even though they are often not the staff's actual employer. The rest of the staff will meekly submit to a lecture about an alleged mistake on their part, whereas they must find some discreet way to bring the physician's mistakes to his attention so as not to offend him. ("Uh, Dr. Hilfiker, could we slow Mrs. Ringley's IV down a bit? She had to urinate every thirty minutes last night.") Serious mistakes on the part of the physician are not talked about except, perhaps, behind his back.

Many of the best nurses I knew did not stay in regular hospital or office nursing. Of the younger nurses on our small hospital staff, three left to become public health nurses a field where, among other attractions, there is much more independence, one left to go to medical school, and a number of others simply chose to leave nursing altogether. There was frequent talk of going back to school to become a nurse practitioner or anesthetist, of going overseas where one's skills would be utilized to a greater extent.

The degeneration of the physician-staff relationship into authoritarianism has a long and glorious history. In part it stems from the physician's habit of relating to patients in an authoritarian fashion. The habit simply generalizes to other relationships. The physician's high level of expertise also contributes to this attitude. There is often the unspoken assumption that he knows the job of each team member better than that team member himself. If this assumption was ever true, it has certainly long been invalidated by the high levels of training given to most nurses, technicians, pharmacists, and therapists today.

In part the physician's prerogative derives from his social and economic class. The physician has more prestige and a higher salary than other members of the team, and in our culture these factors go a long way in defining a relationship. Each of the other pressures examined in this book contributes to the physician's tendency to authoritarianism. When stressed, he finds it easier to demand obedience from his staff than to enter into a dialogue in which he might have to face even more uncertainty. Finally, the traditional sex-role division—male physician and female nurse—perpetuates the tendency toward physician domination.

Once or twice a month our clinic office had staff meetings in which we would gather together to discuss any issues of concern. Each of us, of course, had his or her own job to do. Jackie Mullen's as receptionist was surely one of the most difficult. Handling both the telephone and the front desk, she had to make appointments, field questions, listen to complaints, and collect the charges. People who are sick are not always at their most pleasant, so Jackie's job of screening walk-in patients and telephone calls from people wanting to be seen right away was especially taxing, calling for a precise blend of patience, gentleness, empathy, and firmness. Mattie Hackley worked as secretary, transcribing our dictation and keeping records. She had been with the clinic longer than anyone else and knew the intricacies of virtually every job in the office, since she had occupied them all at one time or another. Mirna Jacobsen handled the bookkeeping and the insurance while Dorothy Schmidt filled in wherever necessary. All of the clerical staff as well as Tiffany Tierney, the clinic administrator, Marge, and the other nurse, Gail Brock, joined us doctors at those regular staff meetings.

The process at the meetings was invariably the same. Tiffany, a young and energetic professional administrator hired primarily to handle relations with the federal agency that was partially funding the clinic, would raise an issue that had been plaguing everyone and try to elicit participation. "Listen, gang. The encounter slips are not getting back out to Jackie at the desk. They're getting stuck with the docs. If Jackie doesn't get the slips, she doesn't know what to charge people, and it's real important that we ask people to pay when they're leaving the office. What's the problem?"

Silence.

Finally Mattie chips in, "People are willing to pay at the desk if we tell them what they owe, but we can't do it if we don't have the fee slips."

After another thirty seconds of silence, Tiffany asks, "Well, where are they getting hung up? Who's keeping them?"

Silence. Everybody knows, of course, who's keeping them; but there is an obvious reluctance to point an accusing finger at the doctors.

Finally my partner, Dan Marks, breaks the silence. "I keep forgetting the damn things until after the patient's left. How about if Marge and Gail check with the patients before they leave?"

Marge scowls at Gail. "I do it when I'm here at the desk, but often I'm back with another patient and don't see them leave. Sometimes they've got them in their purses, too, so you don't know. I wonder how many people just walk out of the office and take their slips with them."

"I try to fill those things out, but I don't like them," I pitch in. "I don't like to charge people, I guess, and I'm almost embarrassed by the slips. Could Jackie be responsible for coming back here and reminding us if we don't give them the slips?"

"I can't be leaving the desk all the time. There's too many people out there."

And so the conversation would go. The problem clearly lay with us physicians and would have been solved only by our taking a more active part in the business affairs of the clinic. Yet we were reluctant to do so, and everyone else was unwilling to confront us. After the meeting, there would be little buzz groups with many suggestions for solving the problem, but it was rare indeed that we physicians were called to task by the other staff members, despite the fact that—in our clinic, at least—we were all employees of a community board. Most of our meetings turned out, in fact, to be discussions between the physicians and Tiffany. Once we got to talking, the other staff would rarely take part.

The disadvantages of such a hierarchical structure for a well-run office or for the patient's medical care are clear. No one has any real input into the decision-making process except the doctors. The nurses know that the doctors are unlikely to read their chart notes, so those notes become less complete and less helpful as nurses struggle through the masses of other paperwork they confront. In the end, a wide gap develops between physicians and the rest of the staff, and it is difficult for information to flow either way.

But the most damaging effect of hierarchy may be to exclude the physician from a closer relationship with the staff which might aid in preventing or at least healing the wounds of practice. On a purely practical level, a strict hierarchy of the sort that generally exists does not really allow the "subordinate" to help the physician. When Melanie Ochsling was hired by the hospital as our town's first physical therapist, it had been several years since any of us doctors had written orders for physical therapy, and we really didn't know very much about the modalities available or their indications. Physical therapists receive extensive training in the care and treatment of a variety of illnesses, but they are trained by and usually work under physicians who are specialists in the field of physical medicine and rehabilitation. Melanie was therefore used to working with experts who wrote explicit orders about what she should do. When she first arrived, I explained to her that I didn't know much about physical therapy, and I would appreciate her giving me feedback about the appropriateness of my orders.

Months went by, and I referred more and more patients to Melanie. Patients liked her and appreciated her help. From time to time I would pass her in the hospital corridor and ask if my orders were appropriate, and she would invariably answer that they were fine. I still felt uncomfortable with my lack of knowledge in the area of physical therapy, but I thought no more about it until Mel Jacobs returned to the office saying that the phys-ical therapy I'd ordered for his neck strain hadn't really helped. That afternoon I asked Melanie if the orders I'd written were OK.

"Sure, they're fine," she said.

"Well, Mr. Jacobs doesn't seem to be getting much better."

"No, it doesn't seem to help him very much."

"Any suggestions?"

"Well"—Melanie looked down—" the doctors where I was trained didn't usually order continuous traction like you did. Maybe if I tried intermittent traction, like two minutes on and two minutes off, that would help. What do you think?"

"Hmmm. I've never heard of that. Anything else?"

"Well it would probably help to hot-pack the neck for a few minutes before giving the traction. And you know, the doctors down there usually had us teach the patients to do their own traction at home a couple of times a day. We could try that with Mr. Jacobs."

In the space of a few minutes, Melanie had instructed me in the current treatment of neck sprains. Her training must have so inculcated the idea of the physician's omniscience that she could not recognize her own consid-erable expertise in relation to my ignorance. It took several years of my prodding before she felt free enough to advance suggestions of her own without my specifically asking for them.

For his part, the physician often finds it difficult to step down from his usual place of authority and ask for help. It seems like an admission of weakness. After Mr. Murphy died in our coronary care unit, I was wrapped in a dark cloud of guilt for days. In retrospect, I can see that it would have helped enormously if I had stayed awhile, talked it all over with Ardyce, reviewed the heart-monitor tracings with her, let her know that I was feeling terrible about having gone back to bed after Mr. Murphy's heart- beat became irregular. But at the time I could not do it. In the back of my mind were the nagging questions: If I admitted my ignorance in this situ-ation, how could I expect Ardyce to carry out my orders the next time? If I really broke down and requested emotional support, would Ardyce and the others respect me or allow me to lead? If I candidly discussed my uncertainties about a treatment I was considering, wouldn't that diminish my authority? These fears and others like them may be exaggerated, but I am often too scared or too tired to risk it.

Moreover, the rest of the staff may be so accustomed to an authoritarian setup that a physician's first halting attempts to reveal more of himself are met with an awkward, stunned silence. It may feel more comfortable for both parties to stay in a known relationship than to take a chance. The end result is isolation from potentially healing human contact. The physician is left alone with the overwhelming burden of being helper, healer, doer, of conforming to the expectations of "good men" in our dominant Western culture. He is ideally always in charge, not swayed by emotion (yet com-passionate), efficient, powerful, omniscient.[11] The possibility of sharing is lost, and the physician goes his own way.

If it is a rigid hierarchy that isolates the physician from the rest of the medical personnel he works with, it is the related phenomenon of compe-tition that isolates him from other physicians. The same inner need to be "one up" that leads to authoritarian relationships with patients and other staff often results in painful, closed, and competitive relationships with other physicians.

Elina Jarvinen is an older nursing-home patient whom I have attended for several years. A few days ago I admitted her to the hospital for what I thought was pneumonia, but she hasn't responded to the usual treatment. I examined her again yesterday, but was confused by the multitude of chronic problems she has, and could not define any clear cause for her failure to improve. In desperation, I ask Dan Marks to examine her too.

Even asking him is a difficult step. He's a little younger than I am, but we went to the same medical school and did our internship together. With this identical training, there is no a priori reason why he should be able to solve Mrs. Jarvinen's problem any better than I can. But I suspect that Dan is brighter than I am, and he certainly tends to be more thorough. He will also, I tell myself, approach her case without the biases I've developed over the years as her doctor. Nevertheless, I can't help secretly hoping that he doesn't find anything new.

I come over to the hospital after office hours and find Dan just finishing his dictation on Mrs. Jarvinen. With some trepidation I ask him what he thinks.

"Well," he says, looking at me, "I don't think it's pneumonia. I think it's heart failure." Do I detect a gleam in his eye? "Your admission note didn't say anything about a heart murmur. I'm pretty sure I hear an S_3 murmur, which would be good evidence for heart failure. Did you listen to her heart carefully? You remember she had heart failure back in 1977?"

I can feel my heart beating faster. No, I hadn't remembered her previous heart failure. Dan must have checked her records pretty carefully. And an S_3, that soft extra sound the heart makes when its failing? I don't specifically remember listening to her heart on my admission exam, although I'm sure I did as part of my routine. It's entirely possible, though, that I listened hurriedly because I was so sure she had pneumonia, and it was night-time, and I was in a hurry to get home...I might have missed it. Certainly I haven't listened carefully to her heart since she was admitted. "No," I say, "there was no murmur on admission. It might have developed since then."

"Hmm. Well, I think her x-ray is actually more compatible with heart failure than with pneumonia, though its hard to be sure; and her lungs sound wetter than I'd expect in pneumonia. I think she's probably in failure. That low-grade fever might be from a mild secondary pneumonia, though, so I'd suggest you keep her on the antibiotics, just to be sure. But start her on some digoxin and a diuretic. I expect she'll improve in a few days."

I can feel Dan being gentle, tiptoeing around a possible mistake of mine, but I wonder what he's really thinking. He sounds so confident, so certain. I feel like an intern again. My intellect tells me that pneumonia and heart failure can at times be impossible to distinguish, and that Dan has the added information that Mrs. Jarvinen hasn't improved on my treatment for pneumonia. Perhaps if I'd been the consultant I would have come to the same conclusion, but I feel stupid anyway for not having thought of it before. It seems so clear to me now. I don't feel relieved that I can offer Mrs. Jarvinen a better treatment, or pleased that I had the courage to ask for my partners help; I just feel inferior, put down. It's such a small incident. Why should it loom so large, seem like such a failure in my head? I brood about it all day. Perhaps the next time I'll just blunder along without help, and the next Mrs. Jarvinen will pay the price for the crazy, competitive feelings that are deep inside me and most other doctors.

Doctors are selected and trained to be competitive, and I am no exception. One has to be competitive to survive the premedical winnowing process and make it into medical school, competing very successfully in college to qualify land then half the qualified applicants are denied entrance because of lack of space. Once one is admitted, the struggle only continues, partly because the selection process ensures a class full of competitors, partly because there is constant vying for desirable residencies, partly because the best grades and the rewards go to the student who can, on his own, come up with the right answers. Cooperation seems almost like cheating.

Competition is not the only factor, of course. Other physicians have the same intolerance for mistakes that I have, the same pressure to be efficient, the same habit of clinical detachment, and the same need to function independently. Dan undoubtedly felt the same way about my mistake with Mrs. Jarvinen as he would have about his own. One would think, though, that once we physicians have passed beyond our training, the overwhelming amount of knowledge and expertise required would ensure cooperative relationships among us; but we inhibit ourselves from entering into those relationships because of the habits of our training and the stresses of our work. The pressure to perform, to be the best, continues and undermines the attempts to cooperate closely.

In our own small clinic we even worked actively to overcome our competitive tendencies. We learned, despite the pain, to ask each other for help on difficult cases. We each developed areas of special expertise which would be available to the others. We shared a call schedule and saw each other's patients. Despite all this, we rarely talked about our mistakes and how they left us feeling. We found it difficult to support one another's attempts to deal with the pressures of being physicians. However much we may have wanted to be of help to one another, we couldn't really cooperate except in a momentary and crippled fashion, couldn't really reach out to each other, much less take the harder step of reaching out to those "below" us. We were still alone with our problems, like so many of the patients we were trying to heal.

Chapter 13

MONEY

"HOW MUCH DO I OWE you, Dr. Hilfiker?" Mrs. Simpson reaches for her pocketbook. "I'm so grateful you were available; you've been wonderful with Justin."

"Oh, don't worry about it now. We'll bill you later." I'm surprised how much my feelings have changed. An hour ago when the phone awakened me at home and Grace Maki summoned me to the emergency room to suture six-year-old Justin Simpson's lacerated lip, I was tired and resentful at being dragged out in the middle of the night. By the time I drove down to the hospital and introduced myself to the Simpsons, I could at least behave reasonably. Now, at 3:00 A.M., I'm actually feeling good. Justin has been a perfect patient. He'd apparently fallen off the top of his cousin's bunk bed during the middle of the night and had a nasty cut, but he lay quietly and patiently under the sterile drape as I injected the local anesthetic into his lip and sewed it up. The repair took longer than usual since the cut was deep, and I put stitches in under the skin to hold the tissue together. I also had to use very fine stitches on the skin and put them quite close together in order to minimize the scarring. But I've always enjoyed suturing lacerations, and Justin's repair looks pretty good. I can be proud of my work.

I take off my surgical gloves and blow one of them into a giant balloon, paint on a grotesque face with Magic Marker, and hand it to Justin—my favorite kid-pleaser. Grace is just wiping the dried blood from his face, but Justin takes the balloon and beams toward his mother.

Everybody is happy.

Mrs. Simpson rummages through her pocketbook. "Well, I'd really rather pay you right now. Were from out of town, you know, just visiting my sister. We kind of like to pay as we go. Things are always a little tight with us, so if I don't pay you now, you may never get it. How much do I owe you?"

"I'm not really sure," I say, avoiding her eyes. I'm suddenly uncomfortable. I'm always uncomfortable when the subject of fees comes up. It's true that I don't know what she owes me since I've avoided learning the fee schedule, but I suspect the bill for my services alone will be over $150. Surgical procedures are always charged at a high rate, and suturing on the face is especially expensive. Those four extra stitches under the skin—the "layering technique" used to decrease the amount of scarring but not absolutely essential to adequate healing—probably doubled the cost of the procedure. And night calls are especially expensive. It's going to be costly. "I'm not really sure," I repeat, staring at the prescription pad in my hands. "Our bookkeeper at the clinic takes care of all that. There'll be a bill from the hospital, too, for the use of the emergency room, but there's nobody here right now who could take your check. Why don't we just bill you? We trust you." I smile weakly.

She stops looking through her purse. "Well, OK. I'm very grateful to you. I never expected to get such good service up here, uh, so far away from things. But my sister said there'd be someone available right away. Thank you very much."

I'm embarrassed. She's not going to be so grateful when she sees the bill. There'll be about $50 for the emergency room plus our bill, a total of probably over $200. All for forty-five minutes of stitching up a lip. I never even asked her if she wanted to pay for the extra layering, because I assumed she had insurance. How much do the Simpsons make? Can they afford all of this? The questions whirl through my mind, but all I say is "Sure, you're welcome. That's what we're here for. Call over to the office tomorrow to make an appointment with me for Friday so I can take the stitches out. You can talk with Mirna, our bookkeeper, about the bill then if you want to."

Mrs. Simpson bundles Justin up and they leave the hospital. Grace begins to clean up the emergency room. I dictate a brief note on what I did and head up the hill.

The financial rewards of working as a physician in America are obvious. Yet, at least in my own mind, there is a confusion within medicine about money. Doctors' salaries are several times those of other medical workers; fees are arbitrary and often irrationally high; the cost of medical care is a significant barrier to many people. The relative wealth of physicians in comparison with their patients often aggravates the stresses of trying to provide personal, caring medical attention; and the desire to maintain a high economic status often interferes with physicians' efforts to ameliorate the intrinsic stresses in their work. Rarely mentioned within the consulting room, money is a subject that too frequently confuses both physician and patient.

Although physicians and other medical personnel work about the same number of hours—the average for physicians is about fifty hours per week, according to the American Medical Association—physicians earn from two to ten times as much as their co-workers. In our office, about 45 percent of the fee a patient paid was allocated to the physician as wages and benefits. The remaining 55 percent paid the salaries of the nurses, clerical staff, administrator, and maintenance person and covered the overhead: purchase of the building, equipment, and supplies; continuing education for the nurses and physicians; malpractice insurance; utilities; and so on. When I left the practice in the spring of 1982, I was earning a little over $40,000 a year, more than twice Marge's salary and over three times the salaries of Jackie, Mattie, Mirna, and the others who worked on the clerical side of the office. Most physicians' offices are private businesses owned by the physicians themselves. Although ours was a nonprofit corporation owned and directed by a board elected from the community, physicians' salaries were comparable to (though somewhat lower than) salaries of physician-owners in the same area.

I thought about our salary differentials frequently. Certainly, I worked slightly longer hours than Marge did, and yes, I did have the added stress of being on call. But Marge too was a trained professional who took a great deal of personal initiative and responsibility for patient care.

She too worked unpaid overtime when patients ran late or there was extra work to do. The magnitude of the difference in our salaries didn't make sense.

The charges made to patients were even more difficult to understand. The fee schedule remains for me a tangle of arbitrariness despite my attempts to understand it. The basic charges for different kinds of visits (brief, intermediate, extended, and complete evaluation) are fairly straightforward. When I left, we were charging $20 for an intermediate visit (the most common, routine office visit) and up to $50 for a complete evaluation, not including laboratory or x-ray costs. But there are no clear criteria for what constitutes which kind of visit, and there is plenty of leeway (by changing the category) for charging more or less depending on the patient's financial status, the mood of the doctor, or the tenor of the consultation. Even for these common and basic visits, then, the patient can never be sure in advance how much he will be charged.

If charges for routine visits are difficult to predict, charges for procedures become a labyrinth of arbitrary rates almost independent of the time involved. A "procedure" is anything the physician does to the patient— suturing lacerations, withdrawing fluid from a swollen joint, performing a proctoscopy, operating on an appendix. I could charge up to $60 an hour for time talking with a patient about his severe emotional problems, but if I entered the surgery suite and performed an appendectomy during that same hour, I could charge well over $400.

The rationale behind these huge differentials is supposed to be the difference in skill and "intensity" involved, a rationale that makes no sense at all to anyone who has first counseled a person with severe emotional problems and then gone into the next room to sew up a laceration like Justin Simpson's. In fact, the fee schedule is oriented around what "third-party payers"—insurance companies, Medicaid, Medicare, and so forth—have historically been willing to pay for particular services. The resulting hodgepodge of fees is incomprehensible to anyone trying to understand the system rationally. As a consequence, patients can have little idea of what to expect on their bill unless they know in advance exactly what is to be done to them and ask specifically about the fees. Even then, they will frequently be told that the doctor can't be sure what will be done and that the bill may vary.

The reasons physicians' fees are so high and physicians so well paid can be understood only by describing the history of American medicine—a task beyond my abilities or purposes here. Suffice it to say that the high salaries physicians earn are not intrinsic to what we do, as evidenced by the fact that in many other Western countries physicians earn salaries more commensurate with those of other professionals like nurses, teachers, clergymen, and lawyers. The high physician fees in this country have had more to do with the ability of physicians to organize themselves through their professional organizations, to restrict competition from nonphysician practitioners, and to keep the government from interfering with their fee schedules; as well as with the structure of third-party payers who cover most of the bills. According to the American Medical Association, the average physician income in 1983 was $105,000, over five times the median American income.

These high salaries are reflected directly in physician fees. Between 40 and 60 percent of an office fee goes to the physician's personal income, depending on the specialty, the size of the office, and the amount of that income. Reducing physician income by 50 percent to an average of $50,000 yearly would thus reduce the average fee by about 25 percent, even without doing anything else.

These inflated salaries and their effect on fees underscore the obvious, yet seldom discussed, tension between the physician as entrepreneur and the physician as servant. Although the average physician's ability to generate such high income developed only in this century, the tension is not new: it can be seen in the contrast between the Greek, Hippocratic view that "medicine is a skill so rare that it can be sold at a great price" and the medieval, monastic ideal that the "care of the sick is a duty of charity," that "altruism and medical care are bound in a moral covenant."[12]

It is a Saturday afternoon in late fall. The tourist season is over, and I've been able to finish hospital rounds and see the few patients in the emergency room by noon, so I return home. The pure blue of the sky, the crisp coolness of the Minnesota sunshine, the smell of approaching winter, lure me outdoors to chop wood. I've just begun when Marja calls from the doorstep that there is somebody in the emergency room. I come inside, wash, change clothes, and drive down to see George Wilson, who has lacerated himself chopping wood at home.

"It's just a scratch, Doc. I was lucky. The axe was sharp, but I just nicked myself. I wouldn't of come in, but Margie thought I needed a tetanus shot. Why dontcha just put a bandage on it an' give me a shot?"

Megan Terry, the nurse on emergency-room duty today, has already cleansed the wound and opened the suture tray of instruments for me, but George has a point. The cut is only an inch long, fairly shallow and has sharp, clean edges. It's not over a joint where it will get stretched, so it might just heal without sutures. I'm not sure. I try to be objective, but I am aware of another issue: the charges. If I simply explain the situation to George and have Terry bandage the wound and administer the tetanus shot, the office will charge the $20 intermediate visit plus a $10 "off hours" emergency-room surcharge of which I will get 40 percent. Counting the time I've taken to wash, change, drive to the hospital and back, dictate a note, I will have spent almost an hour on the visit. It would take me only ten minutes more to suture the wound, but the charge would then be $50 plus the surcharge. It's not a question of lying to George or of performing an unnecessary procedure. It's a judgment call, and I find it difficult to remain neutral. George even has good insurance coverage, so the decision won't affect him directly.

"I don't know, George, you might get away with it. It's in a pretty safe location on your leg, so it might heal OK without stitches, but it would take longer to heal that way. There's always the slight danger of infection, too. It'd be simple enough to put in the stitches now, and then you wouldn't have to worry about it."

"Why don't we just put a bandage on it, Doc? I wouldn't of even come in if it hadn't been for the shot."

"I guess we can go either way, George. I'll leave it up to you. If we leave it open, there'll probably be a bit bigger scar, it'll take longer to heal, and it might get infected, but it'll probably be OK in the end. If we put the stitches in, it'll heal faster and you can get right back to work. Won't have to worry about keeping it dry either, once the stitches are in."

"Well, all right. I'll leave it up to you. Why don't ya put the stitches in? I guess I don't want to monkey with it."

George gets his stitches. I haven't been guilty of any great trespass, but I know how I have slanted my words.

Wealth is another way of dealing with the difficulties involved in being a physician. Not only does money allow one the pleasures of our culture, not only does it confer prestige and position within the community, but it also allows one to buy time, to erect barriers between the demands of work and one's own self. With my salary more than twice as big as the average in our county, we could pay for baby-sitting and dinners out, afford vacation trips to get away from town. When I went to conferences or educational seminars, I stayed at first-class hotels and took the most rapid transportation. Money created time for leisure: I could pay for repairs on the house rather than doing them myself, assure myself of a reliable car rather than run the risk that an older, less expensive one would break down. Money was helpful in combatting some of the stresses of my work.

At the same time, the economic structure of medical practice aggravates other stresses and renders them even more impervious to change. High fees and high physician income affect the nature of the physician-patient relationship in profound ways. Patients' expectations of physician perfection, for instance, are intensified by the physician's wealth and class standing and by the expense of medical evaluation. It is difficult for Carl Fitch to receive a $95 physician charge (for a complete evaluation and several follow-up visits), a $35 x-ray fee, and a bill totaling hundreds of dollars for laboratory tests and then to be told that his debilitating illness "might be a virus"…especially if the medical bills total more than several weeks of his income. Yet few patients will explicitly express their hostile feelings about a physician's wealth; they have come to expect that the fees they pay will bring them a degree of certainty that is usually not obtainable.

Similarly, it seems obvious to me that there is a direct connection between the high salaries of American physicians and the astronomical incidence of malpractice suits and the size of malpractice judgments. Both salaries and malpractice rates are much higher in the United States than in any other developed country. Surveys have shown that patients are more likely to sue physicians whom they believe to be uncaring or unsympathetic, and high physician fees are perceived as a clear manifestation of that lack of caring. Although the fear of malpractice has not been for me the worst aspect of making a mistake, the specter of a suit adds one more emotionally exhausting factor to the pain of having wasted someone's money, caused suffering, or injured another human being.

As the driving force behind the movement for efficiency and productivity, money is, in fact, the mortar holding together the whole system. In the last thirty years, medicine has been "monetarized";[13] that is, everything has been given a price tag and subjected to economic analysis. Whereas a significant proportion of medical care delivered forty years ago was "charity work" hospitals were largely supported by charity, physicians often gave one or two half-days a week to seeing "public" or "clinic" patients, and many physicians routinely wrote off large portions of their fees for indigent patients, medicine today speaks much more the language of business, with cost/benefit analyses, time management, and financial profiles being an important part of any practice.

How then could money not significantly affect the way we physicians relate to our patients and co-workers? Even at the simplest level, I noticed myself becoming less sensitive to the economic realities of those less wealthy than I. Having personally the best medical insurance, a substantial savings account, and money to spend on pure luxuries, I had to struggle to remember that the $20 prescription, the $15 return appointment, or the cost of following the advice I offered might represent barriers to health care even for middle-class patients. When Meredith Heasley brought her two boys in for their constant colds and we discovered together how difficult it was for Meredith to cope with her cabin fever and isolation, I suggested that she and her husband get a baby-sitter and go off for several days by themselves. Meredith looked at me incredulously! Hiring a baby- sitter for an evening was a major expense for them, to say nothing of the expense of "going off for several days." I simply did not live with her realities and so was sometimes tempted to treat my patients' financial concerns as childish preoccupations. The economic gulf that separated us exacerbated my tendency to detach myself clinically from my patients, and to deal solely with the technical aspects of their medical problems since their financial realities were so different from mine.

The effect of all this on me is clear enough in retrospect. The fee schedule had made procedures much more lucrative than in-depth interviews, counseling sessions, or time taken to comfort a hospitalized patient. There were also many important services I performed which had no charge attached whatsoever: returning telephone calls about a child's fever, giving emotional support to a family after a death, going to medical staff meetings, to mention only a few. But despite my conscious disagreement with many of the values assigned by price, I noticed that surgery, procedures, hospital admissions, and emergency-room work slowly became a more and more important part of my practice. Dealing with emotionally hurting patients, taking time to educate patients about the course of their disease and the nature of their treatment, even obtaining a comprehensive interview history, became less central. Not that I consciously changed my routines; but money had powerful ways of bending my perceptions.

In addition, the desire to maintain my financial position inhibited many of the changes that might have made my work more tolerable. One response to the intensity of medical practice, to the need to be constantly available, and to the demand to know more would have been to add more physicians or physician assistants to the practice. An extra person could be on backup call at any time to help with a Mr. Murphy and his heart attack or to share the anguish of a Ricky Meier's drowning. An assistant could be hired to cover the evening and night telephone calls, the emergency room, and the routine problems of hospitalized patients. With more physician time available for the same number of patients, I could have taken longer with my patients, dealt with their problems in a more leisurely fashion, looked up information or consulted with my partners about problems I faced. Yet in our situation, extra help could not be hired without reducing our incomes. Third-party payers would not have accepted higher charges, and our clinic operation was already as efficient as we could make it, so the only alternative would have been to lower physician salaries. Despite the enormous pressure each of us was feeling in our work, we never seriously considered that option.

It is not an exaggeration to say that money seeped into every crack in my life. Much of my embarrassment over wealth, however, did not stem directly from our own situation in our little town. We, after all, had significantly lower salaries than the average physician; we had, to some degree, worked with the issue of money and tried to neutralize its power; we had a sliding scale of fees providing discounts for poorer patients; and we turned no one away who could not pay. My embarrassment came more from being part of a medical system that had priced itself out of the range of many. I was aware of the $100,000 average physician salary, of a system which—largely because of the monetarization of medical care—values expensive technology over personal attention. I knew that many in our country have difficulty receiving adequate health care and that medical costs add significantly to the suffering of those already ill. I was angry at having to be a part of that system, to experience guilt by association.

I can see Melvin Anderson angling across the street to catch me. It is Saturday morning, and I'm rushing around town trying to collect a few last-minute items before we leave on our week's vacation. I'm late as usual and feeling pressed for time. I try to ignore Melvin, but he's heading right for me.

"Morning, Doc. I'm glad I found you. That medicine you gave me is making me sick. I've been feeling nauseated, and look at this rash. Came up yesterday at the lake. Itches so bad I could hardly sleep. What do you think?"

Melvin had been in to see me a few days before, and I diagnosed prostatitis and gave him some tetracycline, an antibiotic. His rash looked typical of the phototoxic reaction that sometimes happens with tetracycline: the skin becomes sensitive to light, and exposure to the sun creates a blistering, scaling, uncomfortable rash. "You're not allergic to any medicines, are you?" I ask.

"No, I told you in the office. Never had any trouble before."

"Are you taking any other medicines, anything over the counter?"

"Well, you know, I take aspirin for my arthritis, and I've had a cold so I've been taking some cough medicine Julie had. I don't know what the name of it is. Nothing else."

My mind is leaping ahead. I know this seems like a simple problem to Melvin, and to some extent it is. But it is going to take me five minutes more of questioning to make sure there aren't any other factors involved, another five or ten to drop in at the clinic on my way home and write out a prescription, and still a few more to dictate a brief note into Melvin's chart. Pressed for time, I resent this intrusion. But Melvin probably can't be seen any more this morning by my partner who is working at the office, so the only other way would be an emergency-room visit, pretty expensive for a drug reaction. So I plunge ahead, finishing my questions.

"I think you're right," I finally say. "It looks like a reaction to that tetracycline. Stop the medicine, and keep the sun off your skin for the next couple of days. I'll leave a prescription at the nurses' station at the hospital for another antibiotic for your prostate infection and some cream for the rash. It'll subside in a few days."

"Thanks a lot, Doc. Just send me a bill."

"No, that's all right. Don't worry about a bill. Just stop by and pick up that prescription from the hospital. Stop by at the office when I get back and let me know how it worked out." Melvin and I part.

Why didn't I want to charge him? Why did I feel so uncomfortable when he mentioned the bill? Part of it, I suppose, was that I didn't want to have one more thing to worry about as I tried to get ready for vacation, one more stop to make in order to leave a note on Mirna's desk to bill Melvin. But more important, I felt that tension between the Greek and the medieval ideals, between self-interest and altruism. I want to see myself as the selfless physician serving my patients solely in order to help them. So money is removed as far as possible from the physician-patient relationship. Jackie at the front desk or Mirna through her billing collects the fees. It is a separate matter, different from the rendering of medical services. Money becomes almost taboo, not permissible to mention within the bounds of the physician-patient relationship.

Like the medieval monastic practitioners, many (I think even most) of us physicians entered medicine with the desire to serve our patients, to be altruistic healers sacrificing ourselves for their good. Clearly, even the servant should be paid for working, so there is nothing contradictory between some remuneration and our calling. Yet as the profession has become wealthier and wealthier, a contradiction has arisen. As we physicians accumulate wealth, as we earn more than we really need, we become entrepreneurs and can no longer hang on to our perception of ourselves as servants. Yet we are not willing to let it go, either, to embrace the Hippocratic ideal of self-interest. So money becomes for us the hub of a very serious contradiction. At some hardly conscious level, my income proved paradoxically to be little more than an additional drain on my energies.

Chapter 14

MOVING ON

ONE SUMMER IT FINALLY happened. I knew I had to leave medicine. Marja had gone to Oregon for a seven-week continuing education course to maintain her teaching certification, and I was home alone with the children, trying to juggle the demands of the tourist season and full-time fatherhood. There was no single precipitating event, but I knew I could not continue. Each day I seemed to resent more and more the small things, like the phone calls when I was not officially on call. Some evenings I even noticed myself trying to avoid going down to the emergency room to see a patient when I was on call. I focused increasingly on how much I didn't know, and wondered why my partners seemed to function so competently. I fantasized that they were concerned about my ignorance and lack of skill. The time pressures under which I worked bore down on me and filled each day with seemingly unbearable tension.

As far as I know, I was still functioning well, but the work was clearly getting to me. Marja's absence during those seven weeks meant more than the burden of extra housework and additional demands from the kids. It meant that there was no one around to listen to me let off steam, to help me deal with the conflicting feelings with which I returned every day from the office and hospital, to share my sense of isolation. Over those weeks, the emotional cauldron bubbled until at last it was obvious, even to me, that something had to be done. I simply was not enjoying the practice of medicine, and I was losing ground in the struggle to cope. I could not remain in this work unless I could figure out a better way to deal with its stresses and conflicts.

What had happened? To some extent I had a case of simple professional burnout, a common enough occurrence in our society. There was, however, a deeper pain. I sensed my work was changing my values in ways I could not control. Clinical detachment, efficiency and productivity, prestige, authority, the medical hierarchy, and wealth are all phenomena based on a common value structure in which people are treated as if they were not fully human, as if they were no more than objects to be manipulated. I did not consciously choose that value structure; indeed, I rejected the notion of it, but so much of my life as a physician was spent in its service that it inevitably became mine.

Paradoxically, as I did my best to manipulate patients into conforming to the needs of an efficiently run office, it was I who became the object, the machine. (We used to joke about having to move into "high gear" on a busy afternoon.) I measured myself at the end of the day by what I had produced. I hung on to my authority and power, since they seemed so integral to my work. I certainly recognized the limited power of money to satisfy me, yet since much of my day was structured around charges and costs and since my income level had become emotionally important to me, money was an important value. Patients' diseases and my services became commodities that were bought and sold at a price.

Perhaps the religious concept of idolatry will be helpful in understanding what was happening to me.

> Whatever I may claim as ultimate, the truth is that my god is that which rivets my attention, centers my activity, preoccupies my mind and motivates my action. That in virtue of which I act is god; that for which I will give up anything else is my god. Diagnostically, I can tell what is my god by seeing what it is around which the patterns of my life organize themselves. [14]

So much of my life as a physician centered around detachment, efficiency, authority, and money that I found my own deepest values in danger.

I felt that I might have been able to bear the intrinsic stresses of medicine itself, but I had found no way to deal with the changes inside me. When Marja came home from Oregon, I told her I would have to leave medicine, at least temporarily, at least until I understood better what I was doing to myself.

Marja was not surprised by my decision, only jolted by its suddenness. She had been aware of my unhappiness for many years, and we both knew something would have to change. She, however, had settled into a rewarding part-time job teaching high school German, and the children were securely ensconced in the school system and the community. However, we had talked for many years of spending some time in Marja's home country of Finland, and Marja thought she could get a leave of absence from the school system, so all agreed with considerable enthusiasm to our move.

I consulted my partners and went to our clinic board to ask for a fifteen-month leave of absence—no money, just the guarantee of a job if I should want it at the end of my sabbatical. I knew such a break would be disruptive to the functioning of the clinic, so I was grateful when the board readily granted my request. Board members, friends, and especially my patients were surprised by my decision. Several told me they had had no idea of the stress I was experiencing, and none could identify with my fear of treating patients as objects. I was apparently still functioning normally despite the bubbling chaos within.

Because of the time it takes to recruit a replacement physician, I allowed eight months between my decision to leave and our actual departure. Those months as a "lame duck" were most instructive. Externally, of course, nothing had changed. My hours, patient problems, and daily demands were all the same. But internally everything was different. By embarking upon the sabbatical, I had decided to take my own self, my personhood, seriously. This decision profoundly influenced my experience of my work.

Small internal changes took place. I knew I might never return to medicine, and so I began to see my position atop the hierarchy as something temporary, almost extraneous; it was a little easier to see patients and co-workers as peers. Efficiency became a very low priority. I knew that with no salary for fifteen months our financial situation would change dramatically, so I began to feel less wealthy than I in fact was. As the time to leave drew nearer, patients began to drop into the office primarily to say goodbye, and I realized that our relationships were deeper and more personal than I had known. The intrinsic stresses of doctoring were still there, and were frequently still overwhelming, but I was no longer making them worse with my responses.

I began to feel an uncomfortable ambivalence. I believed I was a good doctor. I could vaguely sense the possibility of a vocation that allowed me my healing skills without wounding me so deeply, but I couldn't pull it all together. I knew I had to leave, but I was afraid I would not be able to return.

For several beautiful summer months, we lived in a cabin on a small, quiet Finnish lake. It was in this peaceful environment—lacking all the pressures of my former life as a physician—that I first began to recapture my sense of self. During this period I also began to take daily time to write about my experiences as a doctor in an attempt to grapple with the issues that had so bedeviled me. What those initial attempts to get my experience down on paper made clear to me was that mine had not simply been a personal struggle, nor was what happened to me simply "my fault"; and I started to dream of finding ways of restructuring medical practice to make life as a physician more possible for me.

At that point, six months into my sabbatical year, I was contacted by Janelle Goetcheus, a physician who worked with a loose collection of inner-city clinics in Washington, D.C. Janelle was part of a small, ecumenical Christian church involved in a many-sided mission to the poor—housing, jobs, child care, spiritual guidance, health care. She practiced with a spiritual community that supported its members in their work together. She invited me to join her.

There was little reason at that time to believe that medical practice would be any more tolerable in Washington than in northern Minnesota. In fact, because the poor are medically underserved, there was every reason to believe that their needs and demands would be greater than those of the patients I was used to, so I could not imagine how I would deal with the return. My feelings, however, ran contrary to my logic. I was captured by the idea of a community of health care providers who not only worked together but shared their emotional and spiritual lives; by clinics consciously founded to provide services to those who did not have them; and most important, by a feeling that I had a calling to work with the poor. It didn't all make sense; I couldn't quite explain it to anyone. Marja, however, understood even without my explaining; she, too, felt a call to the inner city.

Chapter 15

THE WOUNDED HEALER

"DAVID, ARLENE FROM ADAM'S HOUSE is on the phone," Lois Smith tells me as I finish seeing John Pitts for his high blood pressure. It's Thursday evening, our walk-in clinic for patients without appointments at Community of Hope Health Services in Washington, D.C. I move back to my desk, crammed between the machines for testing vision and hearing and the shelves full of outdated medical books, and pick up the phone.

"Hello, Dr. Hilfiker? This is Arlene. Could we send somebody over tonight? Benjamin was sent here on Tuesday from the emergency room at the hospital; they said he was just suffering from mild hypothermia and that he'd be OK, but he looks awful sick. He hasn't eaten a thing since he's been here. Could you take a look at him?"

Arlene Dickerson works full-time without pay at Adam's House, a fifteen-bed shelter operated on a shoe-string budget expressly for the homeless who are recuperating from some kind of illness. Since the health of all the residents there is so poor, I know she would not be calling unless this man was really sick. We have a waiting room full of people to be seen tonight, but the answer to Arlene's question is obvious.

"Of course; bring him over. We'll squeeze him in as soon as we can." I hang up the phone and walk out to the hallway. "Lois, Arlene's bringing somebody over. I think we should see him right away. I guess we should move him ahead of everyone else." Lois is a registered nurse, the founder and director of the health services, a skilled counselor, and a good organizer. I'm not sure how she'll do it, but she will see that everybody who needs care tonight gets it.

Half an hour later I enter the small examining room to talk with

Benjamin Ruffin. It's all so different from the clinic in rural Minnesota. The examining room itself is a former lavatory; the toilet still sits unused in the corner. The donated examining table is missing a cushion, so an old sofa pad takes its place. The room itself, though brightly painted and clean, is so cramped that I have to edge sideways to get around the examining table.

Mr. Ruffin sits slumped in a brown folding chair. He barely stirs as I come into the room. Sixty-three years old, he is clothed in the dark colors and many layers of the homeless—clothes gathered from wherever possible and piled on to keep him warm. I try to interview him, but his answers are vague, and he keeps drifting off into a stupor. "I'm just fine. I'll be all right in a little while"—that is about all I can get out of him.

I ask Lois to come in, and we work to get Mr. Ruffin undressed so I can examine him. His abdomen protrudes with liters of excess fluid, and his liver is enlarged; his lungs sound wet; his feet are swollen to twice their normal size. We have only very limited laboratory facilities at the health services, but Mr. Ruffin's hematocrit (a measurement of the red blood cells) is 22—about half the normal. I don't know for sure what the cause of his illness is, but it is obvious that he is sick and needs hospitalization.

Lois helps Mr. Ruffin to dress while I go out and talk with Arlene. Like most homeless men, Mr. Ruffin does not qualify for Medicaid, at least not here in the District of Columbia, where standards seem inexplicably stricter than in Minnesota. Medicaid would cover his medical expenses completely. He, of course, has neither money nor insurance. Fortunately, the staff at Adam's House has filled out the forms to get him Medical Assistance, a low-level form of government aid that would allow him free access to the local public hospital and free medications from a few pharmacy outlets in the city. Alternatively, Medical Assistance would pay a private hospital $77 a day if he were admitted there, perhaps one-third of the average daily patient cost. It pays nothing, however, for physician services or any other medical costs.

If I send him to the public hospital, I will not be able to follow him myself, since private family physicians are not allowed privileges there. Although Mr. Ruffin would receive free services, he would be attended primarily by resident physicians in training without the advantages of a personal physician providing longer-term follow-up. I am afraid Mr. Ruffin would get lost in the system. Besides, he has already been in one emergency room without receiving any help. I do have admitting privileges at Providence Hospital several miles away in northeast Washington, a hospital that has been receptive to taking care of the poor. Even though it loses money on every Medical Assistance patient cared for, the hospital allows us to admit a certain number every month, as long as we obtain individual permission from the director of admissions. Unfortunately, it is evening and the director of admissions is not on duty. I will have to wait until tomorrow morning.

"Arlene, Mr. Ruffin's very sick. I think I can get him into Providence tomorrow morning. Can you take care of him tonight? I'll call over and get a bed at the hospital first thing in the morning and admit him then."

"Will he be all right through the night? He's not eating anything."

"I think he'll be OK. The only thing I could do tonight would be to send him to an emergency room and hope they admit him."

"No, don't do that. We've been there too many times, and they don't listen to us. Dr. Hilfiker, why did they send him back to us from the emergency room? Couldn't they tell he was sick?"

"I don't know." I pause. I can feel myself caught between two conflicting feelings. On the one hand I too am angry at the emergency-room doctor. He couldn't have really examined Mr. Ruffin two days ago: these symptoms did not develop from nothing in only forty-eight hours. The doctor couldn't have done any lab work at all or he would have noticed the very low hematocrit. One part of me is angry at the kind of care the poor are used to receiving; but another part of me knows what it is like to be a tired and impatient emergency-room physician, to have too many patients bothering me, many of whom cannot even verbalize their problems succinctly; the temptation is great simply to assume that the problem is minor—mild hypothermia. I feel almost protective toward my unknown colleague. The treatment was inexcusable, of course, but I do understand. "I don't know. Maybe they just triaged him out without really examining him."

While Arlene and Mike, another volunteer, bundle Mr. Ruffin back to Adam's House, I dictate as much as I can of my interview and examination in preparation for the admission tomorrow, and write out a set of orders to be carried out as soon as he is admitted. An hour after Mr. Ruffin's arrival, I'm back seeing walk-in patients. Meanwhile, Lois has been busy, asking waiting patients with minor problems or troubles that can wait to come back tomorrow; she shows me the charts of those who simply need a refill of medications and I approve some while asking others to return later for an examination. Despite the hour we spent with Mr. Ruffin, we finish by the 9:00 P.M. closing time.

The next day, I secure permission for Mr. Ruffin's admission, and the following morning I visit him in the hospital. The intravenous fluids I ordered have rehydrated him, and he is no longer stuporous. Like many of the older homeless men I see, however, he is a subdued, beaten human being. His body is emaciated. His eyes stare past me without making contact. His answers are mostly single words, and he volunteers nothing about himself. He simply lies there, a still black body on the white hospital sheets. From what I can gather, Mr. Ruffin was a severe alcoholic for most of his younger life and has been living on the streets and in various shelters for the past five or six years. He has no friends, no family.

The laboratory and x-ray information I receive back from my initial orders does not paint a very promising picture. There is a large collection of fluid around his lungs and in his abdomen; his liver is markedly enlarged and probably scarred from cirrhosis; he is severely anemic. My immediate suspicion is cancer lurking someplace in the chest or abdomen.

Over the next ten days I call in three different specialists who volunteer their time to examine Mr. Ruffin, but we can make no certain diagnosis. One suspects a cancer in the abdomen; another, severe cirrhosis of the liver from alcoholism. Meanwhile, Mr. Ruffin fades before our eyes. His already cachectic body loses more weight. He lies curled in a fetal position. His answers become soft groans. He is too sick to tolerate the invasive diagnostic tests that might tell us what is wrong. After ten days, the specialists seem to have given up on finding a diagnosis. I see Mr. Ruffin daily, but there is nothing more to do. A few days later he slips into a coma, lingers for forty-eight hours, and dies. His only visitors have been a few staff members from Adam's House.

I want to know, at least, what has caused this man's death, but the pathologist tells me he can't legally perform an autopsy without permission from relatives. As far as I know there are no relatives. Our inability even to perform an autopsy is symbolic of the anonymity of the homeless.

As I write this, it has been a year and a half since we returned from Finland and moved to the inner city of Washington. The external contrast between my work here and my work in rural Minnesota is dramatic. I no longer staff an emergency room, deliver babies, or take responsibility for patients in the intensive care unit; instead, I work primarily within my offices caring for patients whose medical problems are generally quite straightforward; specialists are readily available when problems become too complex. Evening and weekend call does not involve long hours in the emergency room or hospital, but only being available to my patients for brief consultations over the phone and referring them, if necessary, to an already staffed emergency room. I work here as part of a health care team and do not feel so much pressure to solve all my patients' problems by myself. I still struggle with the issues of servanthood and money (indeed, the struggle has intensified as I've identified the issues more clearly), but I am reducing my income and trying to place myself more at my patients' disposal. The same basic tensions are very close to the surface, but at least my work with patients is part of a larger whole, which seems energizing.

Each of the clinics at which I work, Community of Hope and Columbia Road Health Services, was founded in the late 1970s by members of small local churches in response to the medical needs of the poor in Washington. Each clinic charges fees based on income, but the income of most of our patients is so low that well over half of our operating budgets must be raised from contributions, despite the low salaries paid to staff and an abundance of volunteer workers. Perhaps a quarter of our patients qualify for some form of governmental financial assistance, but many—including poverty-stricken families with no young children, unemployed single men, the homeless, and thousands of undocumented Central American refugees—qualify for nothing at all that would pay basic medical bills.

We have no emergency room, no x-ray equipment, and only rudimentary laboratory facilities, so patients have continued to use the emergency rooms of the city hospitals when they become acutely ill. Washington, like many cities, has an abundance of specialists, so some of our patients with known, complicated medical problems are followed at various specialty clinics connected to local teaching hospitals. The patients who come to us generally have health problems that are, from a strictly medical point of view, simple.

What are not simple are the social, economic, and emotional problems that complicate their lives. America Rodriguez, for instance, is a twenty-five-year-old refugee from El Salvador. Her husband works evenings, washing dishes in a local restaurant, while she works days as a domestic, cleaning houses. The Rodriguezes have a one-and-a-half- year-old daughter here in the United States; two older boys are still in El Salvador with a grandmother. America is pregnant with their fourth child. During the last few weeks, she has developed severe lower back pain, not an uncommon complication of pregnancy. The treatment is clear: bed rest followed by several weeks of only light work with no bending or lifting. But the Rodriguezes cannot afford to have America stop working nor can they afford a baby-sitter to take care of their daughter while the husband works in the evening. They have no medical insurance, to say nothing of disability coverage. The medical problem is straightforward, but I am frustrated by my inability to work out a compromise treatment that will allow America to continue at her job while still treating her back.

In a city like Washington, top-quality medical care is available in many different places. It is not, however, accessible to the majority of our patients who are poor and have neither private insurance nor public health coverage. Only half of the roughly 3,500 physicians in our city have even registered to care for patients on Medicaid, and of those, less than a hundred physicians see almost all the Medicaid patients even though the average reimbursement fee is $28 per visit. Only a handful will care for indigent patients with no coverage. A large part of our work, then, is determining what kind of medical attention a person needs and helping that person find some way into the system. Once I determine, for instance, that fourteen-year-old Barbara Moore needs to see an orthopedic specialist because of her knee injury, Sister Marcella Jordan, our social worker, will find out if Barbara is eligible for some kind of public assistance. If she isn't, I will personally call one of the orthopedists in the city who have agreed to see indigent patients and ask if Barbara can be scheduled for a visit. If she needs x-rays, we will send her to a radiologist who has volunteered to give low-cost x-rays; and if she needs surgery, Marcella and I will work together on finding a hospital that will allow the operation at lower rates.

Frequently what my patients need is not so much perceptive diagnosis or advanced technological treatment as someone to be present with them, to listen to their difficulties, to help them make sense of their options. What medical care is available to the poor is too often impersonal, rushed, and bureaucratic as public institutions try to respond to overwhelming problems with inadequate staffs and budgets. Our clinics have therefore consciously set as a top priority taking the time to be present for our patients, even if that is not an "efficient" use of time.

Our appointment schedule is only a vague approximation of what actually happens. Keeping regular appointments is a challenge for people who may be functionally illiterate or who may have many problems more serious than their health—homelessness, violence within the home or neighborhood, threatened eviction, joblessness, or even the need to take whatever day's job comes along. The gaps left by the scheduled patients who do not show up are filled in by others who regularly walk into the clinic without appointments. The paradoxical blessing of this arrangement is that while people may still be given appointments, there is much less pressure on me as a physician to hurry along, driven by the need to conform to the demands of a schedule. If someone needs more time than allotted, I can be fairly confident that one or more of the next patients will not show up.

It is obvious then that Columbia Road and Community of Hope are radically different from the sorts of institutions 99 percent of American doctors are ever likely to find themselves in. To many they would seem pathetically small, starved of resources, and incapable of providing the sophisticated medical care that patients deserve. But the other side of the coin is that sometimes only such small, out-of-the way, financially neglected institutions have the leeway to try out new ways of doing things—ways that might challenge too many vested interests in, say, a large teaching hospital or multispecialty clinic. In that sense, being at Columbia Road and Community of Hope is a luxury for me, one that would not be available to most doctors even if they were considering how to change their lives and their professions.

I have tried to show in this book that American doctors, whether rural family practitioners or high-tech surgeons, face expectations from their patients, from their own profession, and from the society at large that are utterly unrealistic on a day-to-day basis. They are asked to be Renaissance men and women in an age when that is no longer possible; they are expected to be ultimate healers, technological wizards, total authorities. (When a physician refuses to accept those expectations and limits herself to areas of special expertise, she is criticized for being too narrow, or for being concerned only with disease and not with health. When she tries to be a generalist, she is criticized—or sued—for her lack of expertise.) Such expectations add to a rising tide of suspicions of and accusations directed at doctors and medicine, as well as a growing feeling of uncertainty among doctors themselves about the nature of doctoring and of medicine in our society. No wonder that—despite her prestige, her salary, her power—the physician today is a wounded healer. Who could live up to such a world of expectations without either crumpling or hiding behind the masks of omniscience and omnipotence?

So it is important to see what the few places like Columbia Road where there is the opportunity to experiment can actually discover, however imperfectly, about other possibilities available for the healing role in our society. Here, at least, is what I am learning:

I am finding it helpful to share my work with a circle of co-workers. Each of our clinics includes not only physicians and nurses but nurse practitioners, social workers, nutritionists, and a variety of counselors. Because so many of my patients' medical difficulties coexist with economic, social, spiritual, psychological, and family problems, referrals back and forth among these health professionals are very common. When thirteen-year-old Bernita Jessup comes into the clinic complaining of vaginal itching and I diagnose a trichomonas infection, my care does not end with a prescription for the infection. Trichomonas is a venereal infection, so it is obvious that Bernita is sexually active. I try to ask her about this, but she is embarrassed and unwiling to talk with me. Is she willing to talk with Bev Lunsford, a nurse who staffs our adolescent program? I walk across the hall, bring Bev back, and introduce her to Bernita. They spend an hour together talking about many of the issues Bernita has not really faced. A week later, Bev refers Bernita to me for a physical examination in preparation for starting on birth control pills. Over the next month, Bev sees Bernita several times, dealing not only with sexual questions but also with the difficult emotional problems between Bernita and her mother. Eventually Lois Smith is called upon to counsel Bernita and her mother in family therapy. The venereal infection I diagnosed six weeks earlier was only the visible, presenting part of a much deeper problem, one which I vaguely sensed when I tried to talk with Bernita but which I could never have uncovered or dealt with alone.

At Columbia Road Health Services the entire staff meets for two hours weekly to review difficult patient problems, to clear up staff communication, and to join in worship. When Don Martin, one of the physicians, became concerned about whether to continue intravenous fluids in a young patient dying of stomach cancer, the entire staff discussed the issue. Sister Marcella, Janelle and I, and several of the nursing assistants knew the patient well from visits over several months' time, so we were able to share our points of view. In the end Don did not have to take the burden of that entire decision on himself, but was able to share it with us.

Another level of sharing takes place within our small group that meets once weekly for four hours of celebration, worship, sharing, study, and work on our health mission to the poor. Within the group the hierarchy is fluid: Ellen Martin, who is a nursing assistant much of the day, is pastor to the group; Marcella, who works side by side with me as a social worker, is my spiritual director. We take a portion of each meeting to share with each other some of the meaningful events of the past week, and so come to share each other's spiritual and emotional journeys as well as our medical work. The issues of hierarchy, prestige, and competition—while surely present— do not totally dominate our relationships.

This is all, of course, far from perfect. Arlene Dickerson still calls me "Dr. Hilfiker"; I call her "Arlene." No one else participates while America Rodriguez and I struggle to treat her back pain, and I deal with my frustration alone. We doctors still exert a disproportionate influence at staff meetings and in decision-making. Our attempts are flawed, but the common effort has changed to some degree the emotional environment, creating new energy for our work.

Another most important change for me has been to make it explicit that as a doctor I am to be a servant and not an entrepreneur. I have begun to respond to patients more on their own terms than on mine.

My beeper sounds on my Saturday morning on call, and I am instructed to call Arlene at Adam's House. "Thanks for calling, Dr. Hilfiker. George Hobart got beat up two or three nights ago, and he won't go see the doctor. His eye looks pretty bad, and I'm worried about him. Could you possibly come over and take a look?" Her question is meek, tentative.

"Well, I can come over, Arlene, but I won't be able to do anything there. If his eye's injured, he'll have to be seen by a specialist or go to an emergency room. That's all I'll be able to tell him." Despite my commitment to servanthood, I feel myself holding back, not wanting to take the time for this probably futile "house call."

"I know," she says, "but maybe he'll listen to you. We've been trying to get him to the doctor for the last two days, and he just won't go. Could you just come over and look?"

"All right. I'm over at the hospital finishing up rounds now. I'll drop by on my way home."

Adam's House is an old single-family house in a rundown neighborhood that a small group of community activists have purchased, fixed up, and invited their destitute clients to share. As I ride my bike to the front sidewalk, several men are sitting on the front step of the house. I wheel my bike up the front walk, and Arlene steps onto the porch.

"Dr. Hilfiker, this is George Hobart," she says, motioning to one of the men on the steps. "George, this is Dr. Hilfiker. Can he take a look at your eye?"

"Go ahead. I can't see much out of it anyways. Those guys really punched me out. Hurts still, too." George is only thirty-five, but he looks fifty, a common phenomenon among the homeless. He sits still while I bend over to take a look.

"Can you see out of that eye, Mr. Hobart?" I ask, peering at the swelling around the bloodshot eye.

"Yeah, I can see some," he says, covering his other eye with his hand, "but it's blurry."

"You having any double vision, seeing two of anything? How about when you look up, you have any double vision?"

"Well, maybe when I look up, I do."

I examine the eye briefly and confirm my suspicion. Mr. Hobart has what looks like a blow-out fracture of the orbit: the force of the blow probably broke the thin plate of bone underneath the eye, and the eye muscle in that area is trapped in the fracture. He will need surgery in order to keep a working eye. "Mr. Hobart, I think your eye is seriously injured. It will probably be OK if you get it taken care of right away, but I think you're going to need surgery. Arlene's right. You need to get over to DC General and get that eye taken care of."

"Well, I don't know. I got some things to do this afternoon. Maybe tomorrow."

"Mr. Hobart, I think this is quite serious. It's important for you to have that eye looked at. Why don't you let Arlene take you on down this afternoon?"

We spar for a few minutes more, and I leave without any definite resolution, but two days later Arlene calls to thank me for coming over. Mr. Hobart did go to the emergency room, and he was hospitalized for the blow-out fracture. Arlene says it was my examining him that finally induced him to go.

Servanthood, however hard to define, also changes the economics of medicine. All of the staff members of our clinics work at much lower salaries than they could command elsewhere. One full-time physician and one full-time nurse volunteer their time without any pay; many others volunteer shorter periods of time. The volunteers and the lowered salaries do more than simply reduce our budget; they also establish an atmosphere within the clinics. No one is working here primarily because of the money: the staff knows it, the patients know it, and our contributors know it. The contradictions have not, of course, all been resolved. The physicians' salaries of $26,000 are still more than twice as high as the receptionists'; given the poverty of our clientele, the gap between their income and mine is even greater than in Minnesota. So there is still work to be done.

Finally, I am discovering that when my work is more clearly tied into the total life situation of the patient and into a team of co-workers, then it is possible to tailor the job to my strengths, to the areas where I can be most helpful, most useful, and yes, even feel good about myself. Rather than expending my energy in the highly charged atmosphere of the emergency room, the delivery room, the surgical suite, or the intensive care unit, I can now concentrate on unraveling the social, economic, and emotional tangles that complicate the lives of many of my patients. Every physician brings unique gifts to his work; part of my new challenge is to discover these gifts and claim them as my own while encouraging others to find their own gifts. The challenge of an unclear diagnosis, a confusing set of symptoms, a new procedure would, for instance, bring out the best in Dan Marks, my partner in Minnesota. He was in his glory with those problem patients; for him it was medicine at its best. I, on the other hand, find I do better when the medical problems are relatively straightforward and I can concentrate on the other complicating factors in my patients' lives. We each need to give ourselves permission to do the work that fits.

I am, of course, still struggling with the same basic tensions I faced in Minnesota. The intensity of my patients' needs, my ignorance and uncertainty, the mistakes and ethical dilemmas, are all still present. Indeed, the point of this entire book has been that these pressures are structured into the very fabric of medicine and present an insoluble problem. My work in Washington is simply an attempt to explore some different attitudes that might mitigate some of the contradictions.

The first step is to allow ourselves to know we can't do it all. Recognizing our own limitations, we can begin to tailor our work to our own individual gifts. Second, we must recognize that we cannot deal with the stresses of our work alone. The hierarchy, the competitive ladder, needs to be changed into something at least more closely approximating a circle of peers.[15] Third, if we are to begin to regain our balance, we must recognize that inherent in the work of doctoring is the concept of servanthood. This is ultimately a mystery: we will always be at odds with ourselves and our world unless we accept the mantle of servanthood along with the role of healer. Finally, each of these beginnings will drastically alter the economics of medicine. Money is the linchpin. Physician incomes must be brought more into line with those of our patients and co-workers. We cannot hope to change the structures of medicine that create so much stress without relinquishing the exorbitant salaries we currently command.

■

This past summer I went back "home" to northeastern Minnesota to visit. I'd forgotten how beautiful it was, how much my soul needs the wilderness, how much a part of me it had become. I felt a deep sense of longing, a desire to be a part of this rural community again. I was almost resentful that I could not also have my life up here.

For ten days I visited friends, went on a family canoe trip, saw former patients, ran the old country roads. Just before leaving I finally caught up with Roger MacDonald, and we sat down to talk for the afternoon. Roger had been the only physician in town when Dan and I came to join him, and he had been our senior partner for the first few years of our practice. Feeling the pressures of the work and wanting to try something new, he had taken a teaching position with the medical school in Minneapolis and spent much of the academic year traveling around the state helping medical students out on year-long preceptorships in small towns. He has come to know rural practice quite intimately both as a practitioner of thirty years and now as a consultant. Since I'd left town, he'd been hired back during the summer to help with the tourist-season overload. Our relationship has always been close, even after he left for the university. Eventually, we begin talking about that unavoidable topic, the stresses of doctoring.

"I'm surprised to see you looking so well," I say. "Summers used to wipe me out."

"Me too. That was one of the reasons I left, but after five years away I kind of missed it. It feels so good when you stop." He grins. "But you know me, I like being busy. It's a good break from the U. Besides I enjoy all the emergency-room stuff and minor surgery. The last couple of years I've learned to ask for help, so Dan consults when the internal medicine gets too complicated for me. I don't know that I'd want to do it all year long any more, but it keeps me fresh and up-to-date for when I go back to teaching.

"You know, I've learned a lot from AA and Al-Anon. Take one day at a time. I think I'm taking a lot longer with patients now than I used to, trying to listen to them, be with them a little. It's a lot more fun for me, and probably better for them."

Roger has found that the very place which proved so difficult for me is now energizing for him, at least when taken in smaller doses. He seems a model of relaxation in a sea of tense, overworked physicians. We both agree, however, that whether in the city with all its specialists and resources or in rural areas with their reliance on the family doctor, it is hard indeed to find lasting solutions to the problems of doctoring in a society so clearly organized to move people in other directions. But perhaps there's hope, not just in small experimental communities like Columbia Road and Community of Hope, clearly swimming against the tide, but also in the stirs of dissatisfaction and the beginnings of new thinking among medical school students, nurses, rural doctors, even academic physicians.

"My students and even some of the rural docs I see on my trips around the state have been stirred up by your writing, David," Roger says, referring to the articles on ethical dilemmas and mistakes which appeared in the *New England Journal of Medicine*. "They're all aware of the stresses, you know, but they don't feel like they can talk about it. Things are changing, though, even down at the U. More and more of the students are looking for ways to be a physician and stay human at the same time. Even out in the small towns, the doctors are more in touch with themselves. Part of it is just bringing all this out of the closet. Nobody really likes sitting up there alone and isolated.

"My traveling around lets me talk to a lot of Minnesota doctors. Over the years I've gotten pretty close to some of them. They tell me about colleagues who are drinking too much or maybe having trouble with marriages or family. It's all of a piece. They want to change, I think, but they just don't know how." Roger is right. A first-year medical student from Harvard wrote to me:

> I have already been horrified by the glaring lack of emphasis in the curriculum on the social and psychological aspects of medicine or the emotional stress of being a physician. None of our professors is willing to discuss the feelings which the phenomenon of disease elicits in both patient and doctor. Only doctors who can provide "miraculous" cures and patients who are cooperative and articulate are presented. There is no time to express our feelings of sadness for the patient, to articulate our fear that he or she or our relatives or ourselves will die, to discuss the impact of our decision to enter a profession where suffering is a constant companion. Instead, we flounder, striving to ask insightful questions both to impress our instructors and to combat our sense of sadness and inadequacy. We are taught from the beginning not to express our emotions, as if they might in some way interfere with our ability to be competent doctors. Conflict is rarely presented; mistakes never mentioned. I often question whether I will be capable of being a responsible physician, whether I will be able to keep up with recent advances, or to stay alert during the long hours of residency and medical practice, or to understand and empathize with my patients, all of which are necessary to provide quality care. My medical training, by ignoring these questions, is not making me more confident about these issues, rather it is teaching me not to consider them, denying me the chance to recognize my fears.

After my article on mistakes appeared, over a hundred practicing physicians wrote me to share their own mistakes or reflect upon the difficulty of discussing feelings openly. Many had already learned the lessons I was just realizing. A Dr. Wellington wrote me:

> Years ago I was covering for another general practitioner and was called to see a frail old woman who had a tachycardia [rapid heart

beat]. Being bloody, bold and resolute, I injected her IV with Aramine [a medicine to raise the blood pressure and thus lower the heart rate], but gave her, by error, ten times the recommended dose. Needless to say, she nearly died on the spot: she became apprehensive, got a severe headache and a blood pressure off the chart. Her heart slowed and became irregular, and she got tremendous chest pain. After it appeared she would live, I hurried to my office and brought back my electrocardiogram machine, which showed signs of a mild heart attack. I admitted her to the hospital, and nervously but accurately told her of my error. I'll never forget the dear lady's words and her sincere forgiveness. She said, "Oh, that's all right, Dr. Wellington. I'll live. You'll learn. Old Dr. Mancey told me that he only killed five patients that he knew of." "Old Dr. Mancey" had been a town doc who had died years before I arrived in the town, apparently an upright and honest man.

My patient recovered and came to see me several times thereafter—why, I'll never know. The doc I was covering that day did not get too upset either, and another colleague—when I told him about it—wryly said I might have done her some good to stretch her arteries and such. (Not that we really believed that, but the sharing and humor helped my awful guilt.)

Roger MacDonald and the other rural practitioners in Minnesota, a first-year student at Harvard Medical School, Dr. Wellington...we are all in various stages of struggle with the same issues. We all feel or have felt the distress and the isolation. Ultimately, I believe, there is no solution to the problem. All of us who attempt to heal the wounds of others will ourselves be wounded; it is, after all, inherent in the relationship. We can try out new attitudes, share the burden with co-workers, free ourselves from the idolatry of money, but eventually we reach the nub of the issue: in healing, we ourselves take on those others' wounds.

Only by recognizing and accepting his or her own wounds can the healer minister to others.[16] It is our wounds that make us human, that bridge the gap between patient and physician. When we have done all we can to improve our situation, when we have created the best environment possible, there will still be the pain that comes from meeting others deeply. At that point we can either fight against the pain, and in so fighting, bring ourselves to a numb cynicism or a fragile despair, or we can accept it, become one with it, and allow it to minister to others.

POSTSCRIPT

IN THE FALL OF 1981, just after I had decided to take the year's sabbatical that would ultimately bring me to Washington, my former partner Roger MacDonald, who still lived in the area although he worked for the University, took me aside for a talk. Would you do me a favor, David? Try an antidepressant!" I was stunned. I was thirty-six years old, a physician who had diagnosed and treated depression countless times, but I had never even considered the possibility that I was depressed. Yet I knew something was wrong (I had ascribed my unhappiness and tendencies to burn-out always to some personal character deficiency), and I knew Roger to be an excellent clinician with a specific interest in emotional health. He had been a father to me all my years of professional practice and knew me as well as anyone. If he thought I might be depressed, I knew I had to listen.

We talked at length, and I finally agreed to a trial of medication. And it was true that I felt somewhat better. But there was no dramatic change. I gradually began to feel better and less burned-out as the spring date of our sabbatical departure approached, but I tended to see my imminent departure from the stress of doctoring (as well as all the positive feedback I was now getting from the community because I was leaving) as the causes of my feeling better and not the antidepressant medication I was taking.

Our sabbatical in Finland was one of absolute joy even though I discontinued the antidepressant medication in the fall of 1983. I discounted to a large degree the possibility of organic depression and returned to my internal explanations that I simply couldn't take the stresses of the usual practice of medicine.

About a year after returning to the States and beginning practice in Washington, however, I became aware again of the stress and my increasing difficulties in handling it. I seemed to be undergoing the same pattern I'd experienced in Minnesota, despite the fact that my medical practice here was undeniably easier and less stressful than work as a rural general practitioner. I decided to talk with a professional therapist. After an hour's conversation, she stunned me as much as Roger had by announcing that she was deeply concerned about my emotional health, felt I needed very long-term therapy with someone, and was at a real risk for decompensating, just as my mother had when she'd committed suicide at age forty-six.

Only after eight years of therapy and several mildly helpful medications was I prepared to believe that I actually had an organic depression. Two further events took away all doubt. In the autumn of 1992 (and the autumn has always been the worst for me) I suffered a decompensation which left me for the first time dysfunctional. While I've never seriously considered suicide, I could hardly get out of bed, could not go to work, could only sit and stare much of the day. It was obvious, finally even to me, that I had a serious problem.

The final proof came to me in the summer of 1995. I'd taken another year-long sabbatical to Finland in 1993 in hopes that the geographical cure would help as much as it had before. While it was good to be away from the stress of work and wonderful to be in Finland, I remained fairly depressed and had a more severe episode of depression in the spring after discontinuing my medications. Once back in the States, I began working in earnest with a psychiatrist to find a medical regimen that might treat my depression. In late spring of 1995, we finally found the proper combination of medicines, and I had a three-month experience of not being depressed at all. As I experienced emotional "normalcy" for the first time ever, I realized I'd simply accommodated myself to a lifetime of depression, thinking that my depressed emotional state was what everyone else also experienced.

That particular "cure" lasted only three months, but it had given me a window on life, a sense of what was possible, and even more, made me aware that I was indeed a "mentally ill person," who needed to take my illness quite seriously. Surprisingly, that recognition was liberating despite the fact that I had already slid back into the low-grade depression I was so familiar with.

My psychiatrist and I continued to hunt for a medication or combination of medications that might work for me, and six months later we found another one. As of this writing, I have approximately ten months of "normalcy" under my belt. It has given me immense joy. The fact that I was suffering from a low-grade (and sometimes higher-grade) depression during all my years in northern Minnesota, however, raises the question of the validity of the perceptions in this book. If I'm just a depressed physician who couldn't handle the stress of medicine, of what value are my perceptions to anyone else?

The image of a mine canary comes to mind. Before the modern era, miners who had to worry about the noxious, potentially lethal fumes that might be released from the subterranean reaches they were exploring sometimes (I'm told) carried with them a canary in a cage. The canary, apparently, was much more sensitive to the noxious gasses than were the miners. When the canary keeled over, the miners knew it was time to get out of the mine or at least find some way to protect themselves from the poison that they now knew was present.

In the same way, I have come to believe, my depression made me inordinately sensitive to the stresses, pressures, and contradictions, *which are nonetheless real*, that all doctors face. I was the only one of my partners to "keel over"; in fact, the practice in rural Minnesota was one of real joy for each of them. But the same realities confronted them and they had nevertheless to find ways to respond.

I have currently withdrawn from the clinical practice of medicine. After leaving Minnesota, I practiced at Community of Hope in Washington DC for ten years. In 1985 Janelle Goetcheus led a group of us in creating Christ House, a 34-bed medical recovery shelter for homeless men. What was unique about Christ House was that while the men lived in the downstairs two floors, we three doctors and our families, several social workers, nurses and assorted volunteer guests lived upstairs in loose community and tried to join the men in their community downstairs.

In 1990 my family and I moved into a large, single family house not far from Christ House and began to invite eleven homeless men with AIDS to come live with us. We called our home Joseph's House and over three years of living there accompanied many men through their last year or so of life and into their death. In 1993, after returning from our second year-long "sabbatical," I gave up my clinical practice at Community of Hope, and we did not move back into Joseph's House. Although I continue to work there full-time, our family now lives in community with another couple, and I now do only a small amount of palliative care medicine at Joseph's House. My primary role there is to carry the vision and to keep the finances straight. I have realized that—given my depression—the practice of medicine is simply too intense for me. For all intents and purposes I am no longer practicing.

While I would certainly give it away to anyone who would take it, my depression has also been a certain kind of gift that allows me to feel more deeply things that others might be only vaguely aware of, allows me to write of things that others might only wonder about. The reception that *Healing the Wounds* has received from other physicians—the literally hundreds of letters I have received from men and women in medicine telling how the book elucidated from them something they had only become vaguely aware of—is further testimony to the value of what I ve seen and experienced as "only a depressed doctor."

For that I am very grateful.

REFERENCES

1. R. L. Casterline, reported at the 69th Annual Congress of Medical Education of the American Medical Association February 9, 1973. Quoted in B. H. Mawardi, "Satisfactions, Dissatisfactions, and Causes of Stress in Medical Practice," *Journal of the American Medical Association* 241 (1979): 1483-86.

2. J. D. McCue, "The Effects of Stress on Physicians and Their Medical Practice," *New England Journal of Medicine* 306 (1982): 458-63.

3. N. Gordon Cosby, *Handbook for Mission Groups* (privately printed). Available from The Potter's House, 1658 Columbia Road NW, Washington, D.C. 20009.

4. McCue, "Effects of Stress on Physicians and Their Practice," p. 459.

5. J. E. Groves, "Taking Care of the Hateful Patient," *New England Journal of Medicine* 298 (1978): 883-87.

6. McCue, "Effects of Stress on Physicians and Their Practice," p. 459.

7. J. D. Sapira, "Reassurance Therapy: What to Say to Symptomatic Patients with Benign Diseases," *Annals of Internal Medicine* 77 (1972): 603-4.

8. McCue, "Effects of Stress on Physicians and Their Practice," p. 460.

9. Sissela Bok, *Lying: Moral Choice in Public and Private Life* (New York: Pantheon Books, 1978).

10. N. K. Brown and D. J. Thompson, "Nontreatment of Fever in Extended Care Facilities," *New England Journal of Medicine* 300 (1979: 246-50.

11. I am indebted to Gwenyth Lewis for this observation.

12. Albert R. Jonsen, "Watching the Doctor," *New England Journal of Medicine*

308 (1983): 1533.

13. Eli Ginzburg, "The Monetarization of Medical Care," *New England Journal of Medicine* 310 (1984): 1162-65.

14. Luke T. Johnson, *Sharing Possessions: Mandate and Symbol of Faith* (Philadelphia: Fortress Press, 1981), p. 49.

15. Matthew Fox, *A Spirituality Named Compassion and the Healing of the Global Village, Humpty Dumpty and Us* (Minneapolis: Winston Press, 1979).

16. This thought, as well as the title for chapter 16, comes from a book by Henri J. Nouwen (*The Wounded Healer: Ministry in Contemporary Society* [New York: Doubleday & Co., 1979]).

ABOUT THE AUTHOR

Dr. David Hilfiker, born in 1945 and reared in Buffalo, New York, graduated from Yale College and then from the University of Minnesota Medical School. He practiced medicine as a Board Certified Family Practitioner in a small town in rural Minnesota from 1975 to 1982, took a one-year leave of absence to write this book, and now works in Washington, D.C., in two small clinics that provide care for the indigent.